God's Design for the
Highly Healthy
Teen

Resources by Dr. Walt Larimore

Bryson City Seasons
Bryson City Tales
Alternative Medicine: The Christian Handbook
    (coauthored with Dónal O'Mathúna)
God's Design for the Highly Healthy Person
    (with Traci Mullins)
God's Design for the Highly Healthy Child
    (with Stephen and Amanda Sorenson)
God's Design for the Highly Healthy Teen
    (with Mike Yorkey)
Why ADHD Doesn't Mean Disaster
    (coauthored with Dennis Swanberg and Diane Passno)
Lintball Leo's Not-So-Stupid Questions About Your Body
    (with John Riddle, illustrated by Mike Phillips)
Going Public with Your Faith: Becoming a Spiritual Influence at Work
    (coauthored with William Carr Peel)
Going Public with Your Faith: Becoming a Spiritual Influence at Work
    audio
        (coauthored with William Carr Peel)
Going Public with Your Faith: Becoming a Spiritual Influence at Work
    Zondervan*Groupware*™ curriculum
        (coauthored with William Carr Peel, with Stephen
        and Amanda Sorenson)

God's Design *for the*
Highly Healthy Teen

Walt Larimore, M.D.

WITH MIKE YORKEY

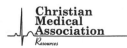
Christian
Medical
Association
Resources

ZONDERVAN™

GRAND RAPIDS, MICHIGAN 49530 USA

We want to hear from you. Please send your comments about this book to us in care of zreview@zondervan.com. Thank you.

ZONDERVAN™

God's Design for the Highly Healthy Teen
Copyright © 2005 by Walt Larimore

Requests for information should be addressed to:
Zondervan, *Grand Rapids, Michigan 49530*

Library of Congress Cataloging-in-Publication Data

Larimore, Walter L.
    God's design for the highly healthy teen / Walt Larimore with Mike Yorkey—1st ed.
      p. cm.
    Includes bibliographical references and index.
    ISBN 0-310-24032-8
    1. Teenagers—Health and hygiene.   2. Parent and teenager.   I. Yorkey, Mike.
II. Title
RJ140.L375 2005
649'.125—dc22

                                         2004017823

Interior design by Michelle Espinoza

Printed in the United States of America

---

04 05 06 07 08 09 10 /❖ DC/ 10 9 8 7 6 5 4 3 2 1

To Kate and Scott—
treasured gifts and now precious friends to your mom and me—
who taught us so much during their teenage years.
To Jennifer, Pauline, Kim, Nancy, Julie, and Kathleen—
who held Barb's hand and upheld her while our children were teens.
And to Bill, Jerry, and John—
who walked closely with me during those same years.

Contents

PART ONE: THE START OF ADOLESCENCE

• What is health? • What is a highly healthy teen? • What role does spirituality play? • The Bible's perspectives on health • A teen's four wheels of health—physical, emotional, relational, and spiritual

• The four wheels of health • The physical wheel: exercise, rest, nutrition/substance abuse, and growth/immunizations • The emotional wheel: love/respect, affirmation/appreciation, media/learning, and boundaries • The relational wheel: relationship with parents, family relationships, connectedness, and performance in school/extracurricular activities • The spiritual wheel: personal relationship with God, prayer, spiritual instruction, and spiritual activity • What the whole picture looks like

• Navigating the explosive growth of the puberty years • Communicating with your teens about what to expect during the physical changes ahead • Staying one step ahead • Suggested ways to get "The Talk" started • The "precocious puberty" trend • The river of hormones now running through their bodies • Learning to speak their "love languages"

PART TWO: THE PHYSICAL WHEEL

• An important teen health issue—driving at age sixteen • Breaking down your teen's growth • How boys' bodies will change in the next few years • Body hair, voice cracking, and even breast development in boys • How girls' bodies will change in the next few years • Breast development, pubic hair, and acne • Variations in the onset of puberty • Physiological changes • "Short stature" children

• Making the transition from a pediatrician to a family doctor • Remaining your teen's health care quarterback • The doctor's role—your teen's health care coach • Understanding the G-U-E-S-T acrostic as it relates to health care • How to find a doctor who respects your worldview and role as parents • Doing background checks and asking around • Getting the most out of your health care plan • The right relationship between a doctor and a teen patient • What happens during boys' physicals • The importance for your teen boy to learn how to do testicular cancer self-examinations • What happens during girls' physicals • Why pelvic exams are not medically necessary during the teen years • What to expect if a pelvic exam is performed • The importance for your teen girl to learn to do breast self-examinations • Why and what immunizations are still needed during the teen years

• Searching for the "cut" look • The steroid shortcut • The truth about supplements like creatine and ephedra • Sources of unbiased testing information regarding nutritional supplements • Couch potato kids • The expansion of obese teens in this country • Determining your teen's Body Mass Index • The principles of good nutrition • The differences between "good" calories and "bad" calories • Eating principles to live by • Fast food and fast calories • Parents who don't cook • The importance of eating dinner together • The latest teen trend: gastric bypass surgery •

What to look for regarding anorexia nervosa, bulimia nervosa, and binge-eating disorders • A pyramid for nutritional health

• When your teens think they're ugly • Building self-confidence and self-image • The importance of the way teens look • When teens want to do something crazy to their hair • What to do about the rising popularity of tattoos and "body art" • Piercing eyebrows, navels, and places you don't want to know about • Fads that are way out there—tongue splitting and toe shortening • Why girls are having breast augmentation • Cosmetic surgery • Clearing up acne

PART THREE: THE EMOTIONAL WHEEL

• The ABCD's of emotional health • Affirmation • Blameless love • Connectedness • Discipline • Six keys to protecting your teens through discipline • Parenting styles

• The rise of rave parties • Designer drugs: ecstasy and GHB • Drugs and date rape • The use of household goods as inhalants • What to say to your teens about drugs • When you suspect drug use • All about Ritalin and Adderall • How a family doctor can help • Testing teens for drugs • The power of the prescription pad for teen depression • Why teen smoking is the gateway to drug use

• TVs everywhere in the house—including teens' bedrooms • Messages broadcast in sitcoms and movies • Why you need to know what's in the movies and videos your teen is watching • Why teens who watch a lot of TV don't exercise and don't interact with the family • Why teens are online more than they watch

TV • The pervasiveness of Internet porn • How today's media cuts into teens' sleep • The importance of rest for growing teen bodies

PART FOUR: THE RELATIONAL WHEEL

• The importance of being a role model for your teen • The link between the health of a family and the health of its children • Why fathers have never been more important • Moms will always remain a strong influence • Healthy steps for dysfunctional families • Healthy steps for single-parent families • Healthy steps for blended families

• Connecting in the family • The importance of family mealtimes • Home activities for parents and teens • Connecting with friends • Supporting your teen's friendships • Connecting through school and extracurricular activities • Connecting with the workaday world

• Why teen sex is such high-risk behavior • Why it's physiologically easy for teens to pick up sexually transmitted infections • The explosion in STIs in the last twenty years • What your teen needs to hear from you about sex • How everyone is *not* doing it • The importance of the father-daughter relationship with respect to premarital sexual activity • The "safe sex" message teens hear in school and in the media • What I say to teens about the importance of waiting • What I say to teens who've jumped the gun • A hot topic: masturbation • Guidelines for dealing with masturbation • What about homosexuality?

PART FIVE: THE SPIRITUAL WHEEL

• The door to a relationship with God is open for only so long • The vast importance of parental spiritual input • Nurturing your teen's spiritual health • The concept of true spirituality • The power of a youth group • Letting teens find their purpose in life • Why Christian summer camps are great • What absolute truth is and why it's essential • The need for more Christian teens to believe in absolute truth • Plugging your teens into Contemporary Christian Music • Making church a "safe harbor" for your teen

PART SIX: TRANSITIONS

• Preparing your teen for the independence and the responsibility of adulthood • The role you should play in health matters when your child moves out to attend college or get that first apartment • When your children go off your health insurance plan • Finding health insurance for your young adult • The importance of a physical before your child gets married • Letting go

Foreword

The contemporary teen lives in a world unknown by his predecessors. It is a global world with satellite TV, the Internet, and much more. Modern technology is exposing our teens to the best and worst of all human cultures. No longer does the homogeneous community environment help us in the rearing of teens. Pluralism—the acceptance of many ideas and philosophies, with none being superior to the others—has replaced common beliefs and patterns as the wave of the future. The school and the home are often disconnected, and the voices from the streets seek to seduce the teen. No wonder many of them have lost their direction.

It's my observation that never before have parents of teens felt so helpless, but it's also my opinion that never before have the parents of teens been so important. More than ever, teens need parents. All research indicates that the most significant influence on the life of the teen comes from parents. It is only when parents become uninvolved that their role of guidance is replaced by the gang, the peer group, or the friend at school. I am deeply committed to the premise that the teen's best interest is served when parents assume their role as loving leaders in the home.

Most parents of teens are sincere. They want to be good parents. They want to help their teen navigate the sometimes troubled waters of adolescence. The problem is, many of them are not prepared for this awesome task. In *God's Design for the Highly Healthy Teen,* parents will find the help for which they are looking. Dr. Walt Larimore is a medical doctor. He has walked with scores of parents through the trauma of teenage pregnancy and sexually transmitted diseases and the devastation of teens entrapped with addictive drugs. He and his wife, Barb, have raised two teens who have emerged as responsible young adults. He shares freely about their own journey as parents of teens.

What I like best about Dr. Larimore's approach in *God's Design for the Highly Healthy Teen* is that he doesn't limit his attention to physical health but fully explores emotional, relational, and spiritual health. Teens are fully human (though sometimes adults may wonder if they're aliens from another planet). As a human being, a teen's physical, emotional, relational, and spiritual natures are intertwined. If there is a weakness in one area, it will affect the teen's total life. Responsible parents must seek to positively influence their teen in all four areas. Dr. Larimore gives us an instrument by which we can measure the health of our teens in each of these areas. After the diagnosis, he gives the prescription—practical ideas parents can use in effectively stimulating the health of teens.

This book is exactly "what the doctor ordered." It's what thousands of parents have been looking for—a practical guide for raising teens. For those parents of teens who want to help their children remain healthy during the adolescent years and emerge as responsible adults, this book will be a welcomed companion.

Gary D. Chapman, Ph.D.,
bestselling author of *The Five Love Languages*,
Winston-Salem, North Carolina

"The Doctor Will See You Now"

Have you ever noticed that these are often the first words spoken by the nurse at the start of every appointment? Something about your teen's health has driven you to the doctor's office. Perhaps he's growing like a weed and his face is breaking out; maybe your daughter is the only one in her class who hasn't experienced a period. Maybe a team sport requires a physical. Whatever the case, once you're in the examination room, you and your teen have the doctor's expertise at hand.

In the following pages, "the doctor is in" for you. I'm here to equip, encourage, and enable you to guide your teen toward becoming a highly healthy teen—so that he or she may become a highly healthy adult.

Perhaps you're holding this book because your children are entering the teen years and you're wondering what to expect, or perhaps your teens are in the midst of the buckin'-bronco adolescent years and you need advice on how to navigate them as a parent. Either way, I'm here to help. I *love* practicing family medicine—especially with my teen patients. There's something about their live-wire personalities and their growing bodies that makes budding adolescents so rewarding to care for medically.

Now I don't know all there is to know about parenting—nor does anyone on this side of heaven. But I do have a few qualifications you should know about:

❖ As a family physician, I've helped hundreds of parents prepare for and guide their teens through the straits of adolescence.
❖ I've reviewed and studied the medical and social science literature relevant to the teen years, gathering the ripest tips for you.
❖ I've studied many parenting "experts," and some offer wonderful advice and others dispense appalling counsel. I've sifted through it to find the best of the best.
❖ I've been there as my wife, Barb, and I steered our own two children through the turbulent teen years, so you can be sure this book is applicable to real life.

❖ And finally, I've mixed all the above with the timeless principles of Scripture. My intent is that you'll discover immediate and applicable help, no matter where you are in your journey.

I haven't forgotten how exciting and challenging the teen years were when Barb and I were raising Kate and Scott. We've been trodding the parenting trail for over twenty-five years. Kate, our oldest daughter, is twenty-six and lives and works near us, so it's easy to run into each other, and we usually share lunch once or twice a week. She is living in her own place with three other girls, paying her bills, and saving something for the future. Most important, she loves the Lord with all her heart, all her mind, and all her soul.

Our son, Scott, is twenty-three and close to graduating from Samford University in Birmingham, Alabama. Scott was more strong-willed than his compliant sister; as you'll discover in this book, he's run into a few brick walls in the last few years, but he has fallen deeply in love with his God. He's turned out to be a highly healthy young adult. I'm very pleased to be his dad.

So while Barb and I feel grateful about how Kate and Scott turned out, we're taking nothing for granted. We continue to pray for our children, asking the Lord to maintain a hedge of protection around their lives. We pray for their future spouses—if the Lord's will is for them to marry—as we have every day since they were six and three years old, respectively. Sometime after our children marry, we might even become grandparents. Maybe then I'll blow the dust off the jacket cover and present Kate or Scott with a copy of this book—knowing all along that it would never have been possible without them.

Thank you for trusting me to walk this path with you and for making this important investment in your teen's health. My prayer is that what you'll learn in the following pages, if you choose to apply it, will help you become a highly healthy parent and assist you in raising the healthiest teen possible.

Welcome to our "appointment."

Dr. Walt Larimore
Colorado Springs, Colorado

Getting the Most Out of This Book

There are at least three ways to maximize the benefits of this book. The first option is to use this simple three-step approach if you need an immediate fix:

- ❖ Assess your child's health.
- ❖ Fix the spoke that's broke.
- ❖ Benefit from immediate action.

Simply complete the wheel assessment in chapter 2, which will help you find the spoke that's broke. Then, using the chart on page 53, read the section that's designed to help you fix the spoke that's broke. Finally, take the recommended action.

A second option is to read through the book to get an overview and then go back to the area of greatest need and drill down. A third option is to purchase a journal or notebook and carefully read and study the book, doing the assessments and considering applications as you go. No matter which option you choose, be prepared to spend time meditating, studying, learning, and praying.

USING A JOURNAL

Using a journal as you study this book can make the difference between good intentions and actually achieving the results you desire. By journaling you'll prioritize what you want to accomplish and make your goals as specific as possible.

Purchase a journal with blank pages. On the first page, write your name and the date you begin your journey toward nurturing your highly healthy teen. Keep the journal with your book, writing notes to yourself as you read. This journal is private—for your (and your spouse's) eyes only.

As you journal, note each principle and the action you're applying, as well as each goal you're setting. Give yourself plenty of time to accomplish each goal. Making progress toward your goals—even if it's steady and slow—is more important than setting goals you can't reach.

USING THE INTERNET RECOMMENDATIONS

At times I recommend information or resources that can be accessed easily via the Internet, but I haven't provided the Internet addresses for two reasons: (1) Web addresses tend to change over time, and (2) I may find better sites in the future. Therefore, Focus on the Family has assisted me in building an Internet site (www.highlyhealthy.net) you'll be able to visit at no cost. At www.highlyhealthy.net, you'll find a list of each of the sites I've recommended. By double-clicking on these listings, you'll be taken to the most up-to-date site for the information or health tools you need.

This site will be updated as often as needed and will host not only *God's Design for the Highly Healthy Teen*, but also *God's Design for the Highly Healthy Person* and *God's Design for the Highly Healthy Child*, as well as any other *Highly Healthy* tools, books, or newsletters that may be developed in the future.

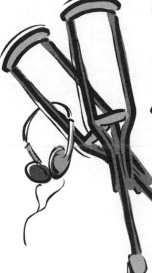

PART ONE:

THE START OF ADOLESCENCE

Chapter 1

WHAT IS A HIGHLY HEALTHY TEEN?

If there's one word that describes the emotions of most parents with children entering the teen years, it's *fear*. Why do parents experience fear? Could it be that before their teen years, our children's lives, health care, schedules, playmates, and values are pretty much under our control? Then, as they pass into the teen years, we realize that, like it or not, their reliance on our direction begins to wane. Just at the time when they're faced with the most life-shaping—and health-threatening—decisions of their lives, we are stuck with the unsettling reality, *I cannot control my teen's life and choices!*

Fear not. I have great news for you. During the teen years, though you have ever-diminishing *control* over your teen's life, you will continue to have powerful *influence*. Once you've finished reading this book and begun to apply its principles, you should see immediate benefits. The fact is, the next few years could actually be not only rewarding but fun!

The teen years rocket by like mileage markers on a long stretch of lonesome Texas highway, and before you know it, youngsters are launched into the college years and beyond. Teens are making critical decisions that will set their direction for many years to come.

The years between twelve and eighteen are perhaps the most crucial season of raising children. They are years when parents have tremendous influence to adjust and shore up the foundation they've constructed in the early years, as the concrete begins to harden. The teen years are the last opportunity to make sure the foundation is the way it should be. If you're afraid it's too late and your teen is beyond your influence, think again!

Let's take a look at two teens—and the power of parental influence.

SARAH'S STORY

When I first saw three-year-old Sarah, two things immediately struck me: she was already significantly overweight, and she was sipping from a baby bottle filled with Coke. At thirty-six months, Sarah tipped the scales at forty-five pounds, which placed her above the 95th percentile range on her growth chart. Most children her age weigh between twenty-seven and thirty-six pounds. Sarah's siblings, as well as her father and various aunts and uncles, qualified as morbidly obese, meaning they weighed one hundred pounds more than the recommended weight for their height.

On this particular afternoon, I gave Sarah the usual checkup and then had a talk with her mother.

"Mrs. Jenkins, I'm concerned about your daughter and her weight problem. As you may know, people who are overweight have a greater probability of having heart disease, diabetes, and strokes. Were you aware that we have classes at the hospital that can teach you how to cook your favorite meals in healthier ways?"

"No, I wasn't, Doctor," she said, but I could tell Mrs. Jenkins was skeptical. After all, many people equate low fat with low taste.

"The classes are held once a month, and our registered dieticians will show you how to cook together as a family, serve smaller portions, and use different ingredients but still eat well. I don't think I have to remind you how important it is to start eating healthier and exercising. Do you exercise, Mrs. Jenkins?"

"Nope," she replied. "We never seem to have enough time."

I took the next ten minutes to explain the importance of exercising more and eating less. By exercising, I didn't necessarily mean pumping iron at the gym. I said that even taking the family to nearby Lake Tohopekaliga several nights a week and walking along the edge of the lake would be a great way to start exercising. I informed Mrs. Jenkins that if Sarah and the family burned off some energy before dinner, it could reduce their appetites and increase their fitness levels. I figured that Sarah was probably watching TV during the late afternoons—a passive activity if there ever was one.

LISTEN UP!

Generation Y is turning into Generation XL.

U.S. Surgeon General Richard H. Carmona

Sarah didn't have to grow up as an obese child. I showed Mrs. Jenkins her growth chart. If Sarah could stay at forty-five pounds through better diet and more physical activity, her age group would eventually catch up with her weight. "And there's another thing you can do, Mrs. Jenkins. You can slowly wean Sarah off the Coke by diluting it with more and more water. All those soft drinks and calories aren't good for her at this age."

For years, I continued to make little suggestions like that to Sarah's mother. I cajoled and pleaded with her and the family to change their heavy-set ways. They didn't budge, so they continued to bulge.

Sarah's first hospitalization for diabetes occurred when she was only eight years old. High blood pressure began at age ten. Her family's inattention and lack of supervision led to asthma, heart problems, and scores of hospitalizations.

I felt sorry for Sarah. She was not only unhealthy physically; she was emotionally unhealthy as well. The schoolyard can be home to cruel comments from other kids, and Sarah's portly physique became the target of barbs from her classmates. "Here comes fatso" was fairly typical, but when the kids asked whether she had an extra Cinnabon in her lunch pail or nicknamed her "Tinky Winky" (after the purple Teletubbie popular on kids' TV), each taunt caused Sarah to retreat further into her shell. She was plagued with a terrible self-image, no inner confidence, and significant adolescent depression. Because of her shyness and the verbal abuse she endured, Sarah never developed any friends at school or in her neighborhood.

Home wasn't a safe haven for Sarah. The one sister she was close to had moved away after finishing high school. Her father constantly put her down and, as far as I could see, never provided her encouragement. "You're gonna be the biggest woman in Kissimmee," he would chide her—not realizing how deeply he was wounding her heart. When I would talk to her about it, she bit her lip and tried not to cry. Sarah so wanted a daddy who would love her for who she was. Even when he complimented her, however, it really wasn't a compliment. "I just love it when you cook chicken good—although that's not often enough!" he might tell her. His love was highly conditional, and she never seemed to be able to measure up.

Her father abused alcohol and usually disciplined her out of anger. When Sarah was twelve years old, her father discovered that she had become sexually active—which proved to me that she was desperately looking for love in all the wrong places. When she arrived home that night, he met her at the door and slugged her so hard that her eye swelled shut. He continued to slap her while she curled up in a fetal position on the ground, screaming for help. A neighbor called the police, who gave him a warning, but after the authorities left, he beat her unmercifully. Hence, Sarah was terrified of her father.

Like most obese or overweight teens, Sarah was considered to be lazy when, in reality, physical activity was much more difficult for her than for normal-weight teens. Her excessive poundage stressed her joints and caused moderate knee, ankle, and back pain whenever she tried to exercise.

LISTEN UP!

The rising ranks of childhood obesity are setting off alarm bells because their numbers have tripled since 1980. According to the Centers for Disease Control and Prevention (CDC), 15 percent of children ages six to nineteen are severely overweight, which puts youngsters at risk for multiple medical syndromes. Elevated insulin levels lead to diabetes, high cholesterol leads to heart disease, joint stress leads to degenerative arthritis, and fatty liver disease leads to liver failure.

Dr. Walt Larimore

Last, but not least, Sarah's family had no interest in spiritual things. They didn't participate in any sort of faith community. When I would raise the topic of spirituality with Sarah, she displayed no interest at all. "If there was a God," she commented one time, "I don't think he would have a single reason to love me." No matter what I would share with her, or how I would pray for her, her spiritual eyes seemed shut.

Finally, at the age of fourteen, Sarah's body and soul gave out. Her last admission was for a diabetic coma that led to a massive heart attack and death.

I was with her when she took her last breath. She was in a coma, and her momma was at her bedside. Her father never visited her during her last few days on earth—but that didn't surprise me since I'd never seen him following any admission to the hospital. While Sarah lay in her hospital bed, I stroked her hair, reminding her that God loved her more than she could possibly imagine. With her mother's permission, I prayed for her, asking the Lord to touch her heart and to heal her.

When I left the room to write orders, her heart fibrillated. We tried immediate CPR, but we could not revive her. When she died, I cried. Without a doubt, Sarah was one of the most highly unhealthy teens I'd ever cared for, and her death was probably my low point in caring for adolescents.

KATHERINE'S STORY

What gave me encouragement was recalling some of the highly healthy teens I'd cared for over the years. One was a bubbly high school student named Katherine—although if you saw her crossing a street, you probably wouldn't think of her as being very healthy. Katherine was born with a congenital brain abnormality that made the left side of her body spastic. She spoke with a bit of a lisp and could walk—but with difficulty.

Despite her disability, Katherine's charming, genuine personality drew people to her, most of whom seemed to love her. For a young woman with an imposing physical disability, Katherine carried herself well and lived a life that was highly healthy emotionally, relationally, and spiritually.

The biggest thing I noticed was her attitude, which was almost always upbeat, and her infectious laugh kept me loose, too. Whenever she would drop something, she wouldn't get mad or frustrated; she'd just laugh it off. Whenever her left hand wouldn't do something her brain was telling it to do, she'd cheerfully say, "That left hand has a mind all its own!" Her mom would tell me how she loved to read and chuckle out loud at amusing parts of the book. She was lighthearted when many who have her kind of disabilities would have been heavy-hearted. Her smile could lighten up the darkest room.

Katherine's caring family provided moral support. Her younger brother doted on her like an English butler. Her mom and dad were Gibraltar-like supports for her, pushing her to try difficult things and always encouraging her independence. They consciously emphasized her unique talents while accepting what she could not do. She was gifted at reading and writing, and her terrific memory served her well in board games. Her parents encouraged her to write and journal. Also, she had several close friends who watched out for her. Whenever Katherine was sick or in the hospital, one of these friends would stay with her or would always be available.

When Katherine was a freshman in high school, several boys began to bully her. They would walk behind her and mimic her pigeon-toed walk. They would call her a "spaz." Katherine would just smile and ignore them. What these boys did not know was that Katherine's best friend was the daughter of the most popular teacher at their high school. When Tina reported the boy's cruel mimicry to her father, he had a brainstorm. He called several seniors— all linemen on the football team—and shared his plan.

The next day, as Katherine and Tina were having lunch in the cafeteria, the bullies sat behind them and taunted the girls. No sooner had two or three caustic comments been broadcast when the bullies were surrounded—and out-numbered—by a half dozen husky football players. The bullies were lifted off their seats and carried outside the cafeteria. The confrontation was not violent, but it was firm. You can rest assured that Katherine was never bothered again!

Katherine's deep faith in God impressed me so much. I never heard her question why God had allowed her to have such a devastating disease. Instead, Katherine would share with me what God was teaching her through her disability. As a young woman full of kindness, gratitude, and hope, Katherine was more highly healthy than most of us.

I've long believed that teens like Sarah—overweight, unloved, and emotionally undernourished—and teens like Katherine—confident, outgoing, and willing to place her trust in her heavenly Father—aren't just born that way. Katherine's mom and dad knew that the personal investment they made would prove to be crucial to a teen's overall health.

What makes for highly healthy teens? Is it good medical care, proper schooling, involved youth pastors, excellent soccer coaches, renowned dance instructors, or good programs like the YMCA, AWANA, and Scouting? My experience tells me that highly healthy teens come from parents who know and exercise their powerful influence by equipping them to become highly healthy adults.

Here are just a few issues you as a parent of a teen are likely to wrestle with in the next few years. As you review the list, begin to consider the huge influence you still have in each of these areas:

❖ How do I assess my teen's health?

❖ How do I begin and maintain conversations about puberty and adolescence?

❖ What is normal teen development?

❖ What if my teen is an early bloomer or a late bloomer?

❖ How do I find the best doctor for my teen?

❖ How much rest does my teen need?

❖ Why are teens so fixed on clothes and appearance?

❖ What's the story behind tattooing, piercing, branding, and self-mutilation?

❖ Why are teens' nutrition habits so terrible?

❖ How do I handle weight issues with my teen?

❖ How do I build my teen's self-image?

❖ How do I teach responsibility to my teen?

❖ Is teen suicide prevention important if my kid is normal?

❖ How do I prevent tobacco, alcohol, and drug abuse?

❖ How dangerous are TV, the Internet, and movies?

❖ What is the best way to discipline teens?

❖ How do I nurture safe drivers?

❖ What if I'm single or our family is blended?

❖ What do I need to know about teen dating and teen sex?

❖ What's the latest information on sexually transmitted infections?

❖ How can I help my teen postpone sexual activity?

❖ What's the deal on masturbation?

❖ Can homosexuality be avoided or prevented?

❖ How does a spiritual foundation affect a teen's health?

Although we'll explore many of these questions in depth, this book isn't a how-to manual or a ten-step guidebook. Rather, the essential principles I'll discuss are designed to be integrated into your daily relationship with your teen.

If you understand these essentials and apply them in your life and the lives of your teens, you'll be better equipped to nurture highly healthy teens in a highly healthy family. But remember that it takes more than knowledge, principles, and skills to accomplish this lofty goal. Nurturing healthy teens requires action. This isn't the time to sit in the grandstands with your arms crossed, watching life unfold for your teens. You need to be standing on the sidelines, much like a football coach, cheering them on every chance you get and sending in the plays that will move your teens down the field toward adulthood.

Putting into practice the essentials explained in this book is—well—essential. To ensure we share the same starting point, let's identify what *health* really is.

DEFINING TRUE HEALTH

Being highly healthy means that our entire being—physical, emotional, relational, and spiritual—must be functioning as God designed us to function. This doesn't mean each aspect must be performing at the highest possible level. Rather, each should be balanced and operating as God designed them to operate. Even if one is out of balance, the other three can become more highly healthy.

In this context, physical health may be the most unimportant component of the four, as it was with Katherine. For teens to be highly healthy, they have to think beyond bodies and emotions; they need to look beyond family and social relationships. They also need to look at their spiritual health.

WHAT THE BIBLE HAS TO SAY ABOUT HEALTH

The Bible gives us clues on what makes a teen highly healthy. First and foremost, the Bible views health as completeness and wholeness. The Hebrew word *shalom*, which is often translated "peace," actually expresses the concept of health through the prism of Old Testament times. *Shalom*'s root meaning is that of wholeness, completeness, and general well-being in more than a physical or emotional sense. *Shalom* conveys a strong emphasis on relational and spiritual well-being—especially one's relationship with God.

The Bible teaches that true *shalom* comes from God: "The LORD gives strength to his people; the LORD blesses his people with peace." King David once wrote that God's way and his peace go hand in hand: "Love and faithfulness meet together; righteousness and peace kiss each other." David's son Solomon wisely taught us that "a heart at peace gives life to the body." The Bible seems to indicate that all people (and this would include teens) cannot be highly healthy physically, emotionally, and relationally *unless* they are healthy spiritually as well.

Another health concept found in the ancient Hebrew Scriptures is expressed in the word *rapha*, which refers to "healing." Various noun and verb derivatives of *rapha* occur at least eighty-six times in the Old Testament, teaching us that God's activity as a healer is not limited to the physical realm. God is depicted as wanting to restore and bring healing in every aspect of a person's life—physical, emotional, relational, and spiritual.

LISTEN UP!

A cheerful heart is good medicine, but a crushed spirit dries up the bones.

King Solomon, said to be the wisest man who ever lived, connecting the dots by relating emotions to physical health

Consider a few Bible stories that describe health in broad, comprehensive terms. David poignantly described the guilt he felt following his affair with Bathsheba and subsequent murder of Uriah and the severe impact it had on his physical, emotional, and spiritual health. "When I kept silent, my bones wasted away through my groaning all day long," David wrote. "For day and night your hand was heavy upon me; my strength was sapped as in the heat of summer." The apostle John also linked our overall well-being to spiritual vitality: "Dear friend, I pray that you may enjoy good health and that all may go well with you, even as your soul is getting along well."

As a theme in the Bible, health is viewed primarily as the restoration and strengthening of one's personal relationship with God, which can be summed up by the term *blessed*. Consider how Jesus used *blessed* in the Sermon on the Mount. Each of his declarations—"Blessed are those who .... "—affirms the Bible's bold assertion that people who aren't gifted socially, financially, physically, or mentally can still be blessed by God, which enhances their overall health. Jesus taught that those who are poor in spirit, who mourn, who are meek, who hunger and thirst after God's ways, who are merciful, who are pure in heart, who are peacemakers, who are persecuted, and who are bullied can all be blessed. We see this clearly in the priestly blessing in Numbers 6:24–26:

"The LORD bless you and keep you;
the LORD make his face shine upon you
*   and be gracious to you;*
the LORD turn his face toward you
*   and give you peace."*

I hope it's beginning to become clear that teens' health depends not just on their physical, emotional, and relational health—as important as they are—but also on their inner spiritual life. Just as a person's abnormal body temperature is one of the first indicators that something isn't right, a teen's spiritual temperature must remain close to 98.6°F to help the body grow in other ways.

What the Bible teaches about health is exactly what the medical research of the last half century has also revealed: without spiritual, relational, and emotional well-being, our teens will simply be less healthy than we want them to be and less healthy than God intends them to be.

Why do I stress this ancient but timeless biblical view? Does it really matter in the twenty-first-century world, where we have access to the most incredible medical technology and health care system the world has ever seen? My answer is an unqualified yes. I've seen many teens in my practice who were healthy physically, yet they were involved with parents or families whose relational, emotional, and spiritual lives were disastrous train wrecks. These families were unable to grasp what it meant to be highly healthy.

One of these families was the McGregors, who had three standout soccer players in the house. Dinner-table talk centered around the next tournament, the chance to impress college scouts, or whether one of the girls would get named to an international team. Sally, Sandy, and Joanie were in great physical health, but their soulless eyes revealed three adolescent women troubled by pressure to win at all costs, to perform at a level high enough to win a college scholarship, and to keep off extra weight. Yes, these young women were highly healthy *physically*, but emotionally, relationally, and spiritually they were accidents waiting to happen. As they progressed into their teen years, they veered off into full-scale rebellion and trouble.

I'm sure that's not what you want for your teens. That's why throughout this book, I'll be teaching you about the four "wheels" of health (physical, emotional, relational, *and* spiritual) essential to high degrees of health. If you want to nurture highly healthy teens, you must understand and intentionally tend to all four health wheels.

THE FOUR WHEELS OF HEALTH

Preserving and improving our teens' health—physically, emotionally, relationally, and spiritually—is our long-term goal. As a family physician, I don't expect parents to have the skills to treat diseases and disorders, but I've long felt that fathers and mothers can be equipped to prevent them. We want our children to have both a high quality *and* a high quantity of life.

In order to understand how to nurture our teens' health, we need to understand a concept taught to me by Harold, who lived in a small cabin near Bryson City, North Carolina. Harold's true joy in life was refurbishing Model T Fords, and he specialized in repairing wheels. He showed me how a weakness in just one or two spokes could cause a multispoked wheel to collapse and, potentially, cause a wreck. If a driver wanted a long, smooth ride, Harold told me, the wheels needed to be as perfectly balanced as possible. An imbalance in even one wheel could put a strain on the engine, chassis, and other wheels.

I began to think about the components of teen health in the way Harold viewed the components of a sturdy wheel: four wheels attached to a stable car (the four health "wheels" of a highly healthy person), with all wheels in balance (all aspects of a highly healthy teen developed in balance).

The four "wheels" of highly healthy teens are:

* **physical health**—the well-being of a teen's body;
* **emotional health**—the well-being of a teen's connection with his or her various emotions;
* **relational health**—the well-being of a teen's associations with parents, family members, and friends in the context of a healthy community; and
* **spiritual health**—the well-being of a teen's relationship with God.

Please take this point to heart: raising highly healthy teens—truly healthy teens—is *not* dependent on physical well-being alone. Highly healthy teens will be those young men and women whose four health wheels are inflated with self-confidence and balanced with parental love and direction.

You may be surprised to learn that these four health wheels were present in Jesus' life. The Bible tells us that, as a preteen, "Jesus grew in wisdom and stature, and in favor with God and men." Jesus grew emotionally and mentally (in wisdom), physically (in stature), relationally (in favor with men), and spiritually (in favor with God). To be a highly healthy teen, Jesus had to grow in all four areas. Your teen is no different!

When the four wheels are working synchronously, parents will see their teens become as healthy as possible—and be satisfied as well. Let's take a closer look at each of the four wheels of health.

The Physical Wheel

The simplest definition of maximum physical health is that the vital life processes and functions of your teen's body are functioning in the way God designed them. For teens to be physically healthy, disease must be prevented whenever possible and treated as needed. What about teens with physical challenges? Those with an incurable illness or disorder must learn to cope and adapt. With good emotional, relational, and spiritual health, even teens like Katherine, whose bodies may not be "whole," can be highly healthy.

The Emotional Wheel

Great emotional health is the state in which teens have maximum emotional well-being. I don't define this as the absence of emotional distress—an unavoidable part of maturing. After all, the swirling of hormones during puberty produces a tempest of emotions. Being emotionally healthy means learning to cope with and actually embrace the full spectrum of human emotions that teens will face daily in their adolescent years.

We will explore how emotional health in teens is founded on love and respect, affirmation and appreciation, media and learning, and well-defined boundaries that need to be provided in the parent-teen relationship.

The Relational Wheel

Relational, or social, health might be defined as the state of maximum well-being in a teen's social relationships—those with siblings, family, friends, schoolmates, teachers, coaches, clerics, neighbors, and the broader community.

Although relational stress and discord are inevitable during the teen years, it is critical to teens' well-being that we learn how to teach them to develop healthy relationships and be diligent in preventing and treating disordered relationships. We'll explore tips on building strong relationships with your teen and look at how your investment of time in your teen will pay huge dividends.

LISTEN UP!

Man must be arched and buttressed from within; else the temple wavers to the dust.

Roman Emperor Marcus Aurelius

The Spiritual Wheel

To say that the spiritual wheel is in many ways the most crucial wheel may sound like religious babble to many. But I'll be presenting some startling scientific evidence of the impact of spiritual health on the physical and emotional well-being of teens. Are you open to exploring a new perspective on nurturing the "whole" health of your teen?

As you are about to discover, if the spiritual wheel receives less attention than the other three wheels, it will be like driving on a freeway with a flat tire. Teens will not be highly healthy and will not grow to be highly healthy adults unless they get equal amounts of air in all four wheels. Just as proper balance and alignment are important when driving a car, balancing all four health wheels is essential to achieving and maintaining a state of being highly healthy.

Consider these words from the apostle Paul, who wrote, "For physical training [the physical wheel] is of some value, but godliness [the spiritual wheel] has value for all things, holding promise for both the present life and the life to come."

For most people, learning to view their spiritual wheel as the one connected to the most important source of power and steering means they can affirm the value and goodness of the other wheels without making them the primary focus of their lives. I once interviewed Dennis LaRavia, M.D., a family physician, who said that true health is a recognition that God is the author of all good gifts, including our physical, mental, and social health. But he went on to tell me that our spiritual well-being is the cornerstone of true health. He was convinced that we needed the peace and joy that comes only from God, because good physical, emotional, and relational health isn't enough to make us highly healthy.

Although the Bible doesn't promise us a perfectly healthy life, God's Word *does* promise an abundant life—one that will be full and meaningful, infused with purpose and joy—to those who have a vital personal relationship with God. Because spiritual health is so crucial, we'll talk more about it throughout the book.

When you understand the four wheels of health, I believe you'll welcome new opportunities for enhancing the personal health of your teen and formulate a plan for taking action when the occasion calls for it. The first step in being proactive is assessing your teen's current health.

Chapter 2

ASSESSING YOUR TEEN'S HEALTH

Here's an easy way to assess the four wheels of health for your teen. This simple tool, though it usually yields only a crude representation of your teen's overall health, will give you a helpful snapshot of his or her health balance—or lack of it.

To begin, either photocopy the simple illustration on page 36 or reproduce it on a separate sheet of paper. (By the way, you can download complimentary copies on the Web at www.highlyhealthy.net.) Use one graph for each teen in your family. I urge you and your spouse to fill out different graphs and then compare your observations. You may also want to seek your teen's input on some of the spokes (e.g., the horizontal spokes of the emotional wheel), just to be sure your observations are accurate.

Notice that each of the four health wheels has a hub and four spokes. The spokes represent the measure of health your teen possesses in each area. The longer the spoke, the better. What I'd like you to do is assess the length of each spoke of each wheel. This will show you how smooth a ride your teen is having.

Please note that this exercise is *not* meant to show your teens where they come up short. (Careful: if they peek at your evaluation, they could be emotionally hurt.) In fact, I recommend you don't show the completed graph to your teen. Rather, this for-your-eyes-only tool is designed to show where *you* need to improve in your quest to nurture a healthier teen. The more accurately you assess your teen, the more helpful this tool will be. Also, let me add that this measurement tool has not been scientifically verified. My guidance

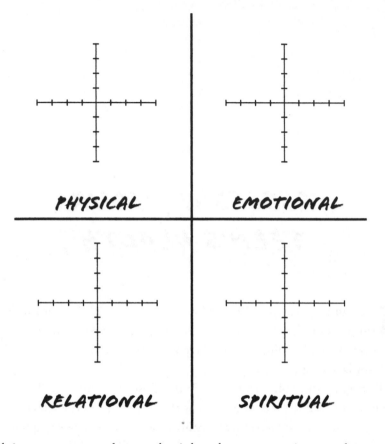

PHYSICAL   EMOTIONAL

RELATIONAL   SPIRITUAL

in helping you measure these spokes is based on my experience and my review of the research literature.

As you read each description below, mark the appropriate spoke to represent your evaluation of your teen's health. The hub is the zero point.

PHYSICAL WHEEL

Hub = trust that your teen's body will develop properly if nurtured
Vertical Spokes = exercise and rest
Horizontal Spokes = nutrition/substance abuse and growth/immunizations

Exercise

This spoke represents your teen's average physical activity over the last two or three months.

❖ Full spoke: My teen exercises (runs, walks, works out, or participates in sports or physical education) at least thirty minutes six or seven days a week.

❖ 3/4 spoke: My teen exercises at least thirty minutes per day, four or five days a week.

❖ 1/2 spoke: My teen exercises at least thirty minutes per day, three days a week.

❖ 1/4 spoke: My teen exercises only two days a week.

❖ No spoke: My teen is a couch potato. He or she participates in no physical education at school and no sports activities.

Rest

On average, over the last two to three months, how would you assess your teen's sleep and rest habits? Consider these factors for the bottom spoke:

1. My teen goes to bed at a reasonable hour.
2. My teen gets eight or more hours of restful sleep most nights of the week.
3. My teen usually wakes up refreshed.
4. My teen has one or two days per week for play, rest, and recreation.
5. Our family, including our teen, enjoys one or more adequate, restful family vacations each year.

❖ Full spoke: My teen achieves five of the above.

❖ 3/4 spoke: My teen achieves four of the above.

❖ 1/2 spoke: My teen achieves three of the above.

❖ 1/4 spoke: My teen achieves two of the above.

❖ No spoke: My teen achieves zero or one of the above.

Now let's turn our attention from the vertical spokes of the physical health wheel to its horizontal spokes.

Nutrition/Substance Abuse

Use the left-hand spoke to evaluate your teen's diet and nutrition habits. Consider these factors:

1. My teen drinks plenty of water daily.
2. My teen eats at least two to four servings of fruits and three to five servings of vegetables daily.

3. My teen eats at least two nutritious meals per day.

4. My teen has minimal intake of caffeine and soft drinks.

5. My teen has minimal intake of saturated fats and highly processed foods.

6. My teen has fewer than two or three fast-food meals a month.

A. My teen is frequently exposed to secondhand smoke.

B. My teen occasionally smokes tobacco.

C. My teen frequently smokes tobacco (daily or weekly).

D. My teen uses any illicit drugs or misuses prescription drugs.

- ❖ Full spoke: My teen does all six of the numbered factors above.
- ❖ 3/4 spoke: My teen does five of the numbered factors above.
- ❖ 1/2 spoke: My teen does four of the numbered factors above.
- ❖ 1/4 spoke: My teen does two or three of the numbered factors above.
- ❖ Subtract up to 1/4 spoke if A is true.
- ❖ Subtract up to 1/2 spoke if B is true.
- ❖ Subtract up to 3/4 spoke if C is true.
- ❖ Subtract a full spoke if D is true.
- ❖ No spoke: My teen does zero or one of the numbered factors above.

Growth/Immunizations

Now let's consider your teen's growth and immunizations. Three-quarters of this spoke is for your teen's growth (weight and height), and one quarter is for their immunizations. Regarding growth, I believe the most reliable indicator is your teen's Body Mass Index (BMI). You can determine this by using the BMI chart on page 126 (or you can access a computerized chart at www.highlyhealthy.net) and then mark the right-hand spoke:

- ❖ 3/4 spoke: My teen's BMI is normal (20 to 24.9).
- ❖ 1/2 spoke: My teen's BMI is overweight (25 to 26.9).
- ❖ 1/4 spoke: My teen's BMI is extremely overweight (27 to 29.9) or underweight (18.5 to 19.9).
- ❖ No spoke: My teen's BMI indicates obesity (30 or above) or extreme underweight (less than 18.5).

You may be surprised I've dedicated part of a spoke to immunizations, but of all the preventive measures for affecting a teen's health, this one ranks right up there. Vaccines have had a greater impact on reducing childhood and teen death and disability from infectious diseases than almost any other public health intervention.

To measure this part of the spoke, determine how many recommended immunizations your teen has received. You can find an up-to-date list on my website (www.highlyhealthy.net). According to the CDC, every teen should be up to date with at least these four immunizations: Td (tetanus-diphtheria), varicella (if your child hasn't had chicken pox or received the vaccine as a child), hepatitis B, and MMR (measles, mumps, and rubella booster, if not completed as a child).

> ❖ 1/4 spoke: My teen has received all recommended vaccines.
> ❖ No spoke: My teen is missing one or more immunizations.

EMOTIONAL WHEEL

> Hub = trust that your teen's emotions will develop properly if nurtured
> Vertical Spokes = love/respect and affirmation/appreciation
> Horizontal Spokes = media/learning and boundaries

Let me point out that the measures I use here assume your teen is not wrestling with any emotional disorders such as abnormal stress, depression, or anxiety. If they are, the measures below are critical for your teen but incomplete. I'd urge you in these instances to seek professional help for such disorders.

You will note that the vertical spokes examine love, while the horizontal spokes examine limits. To put it another way, the vertical looks at relationships, and the horizontal looks at rules. These two must be balanced for your teen to be highly healthy.

Love/Respect

Consider these factors for the top spoke of this wheel:

1. I frequently tell my teen I love him or her. I communicate to my teen that he or she is a blessing.
2. I enjoy talking things over with my teen and try to talk to my teen in a warm and friendly voice.
3. I try to show interest and enthusiasm when my teen is speaking. I pay attention when he or she talks to me—even if it means stopping what I'm doing.

4. I feel emotionally warm and affectionate toward my teen and hug him or her frequently.

5. I feel I understand my teen's problems, worries, needs, and wants.

6. I respect my teen's decisions and support them (as long as they're not illegal, immoral, or something that will cause harm).

7. I look for opportunities to ask my teen for his or her opinion.

8. I consciously look for things to admire, respect, and appreciate about my teen.

A. I feel my love for my teen is most frequently unconditional—that my love is not withheld based on behavior, performance, or looks. My teen knows I love him or her, regardless of how or what he or she does. I do not tie my love for my teen to success or failure in accomplishing a task; to their abilities, assets, looks, or personality traits; to who he or she may remind me of; or to whatever his or her behavior happens to be—no matter how he or she acts. (Of course, this doesn't mean you always like the behavior. Not at all! But it does mean you always love your teen "in spite of . . . ," even when you detest the behavior.)

B. I feel my love for my teen is most frequently conditional—that my love is predicated on how my teen behaves, performs, or looks (love "if . . ." or "because of . . .").

❖ Full spoke: I believe all eight of the numbered factors above are true.

❖ 3/4 spoke: I believe six or seven of the numbered factors above are true.

❖ 1/2 spoke: I believe four or five of the numbered factors above are true.

❖ 1/4 spoke: I believe two or three of the numbered factors above are true.

❖ No spoke: I believe zero or one of the numbered factors above apply to me and my teen.

❖ Add up to 1/4 spoke if A is true.

❖ Subtract up to 1/2 spoke if B is true.

Why do I give so much credence to the type of love we choose to give our teens? It's simple! If you love your teens only when they please you (conditional love) and convey love to them only during those times, they will not feel genuinely loved. This, in turn, will make them feel insecure, damage their self-esteem, and actually prevent them from moving on to better self-control and more mature behavior.

If you love your teens only when they meet your requirements or expectations, they will feel incompetent and incomplete. They will believe it's fruitless to do their best because it's never good enough. Insecurity and anxiety will plague them and prevent them from becoming highly healthy emotionally, relationally, and even spiritually.

A key foundation for a highly healthy teen is unconditional love, which helps a teen reduce the risk for immature anger, resentment, guilt, depression, anxiety, insecurity, and a whole slew of other highly unhealthy factors. Unconditional love balances love with discipline, freedom with limits, and nurture with training. Such a relationship with your teen will be healthy, enjoyable, and affectionate for both of you—which leads us to the other vertical spoke.

Affirmation/Appreciation

Consider the following factors:

1. I am my teen's best cheerleader. I frequently praise my teen and tell my teen I appreciate what he or she has done. I let my teen know I believe in him or her, I trust him or her, and I know what he or she is capable of.
2. I hug my teen frequently and often tell my teen how much I appreciate him or her.
3. I thank my teen for doing things without my asking, and I demonstrate my gratitude for the little things he or she does (even if it's his or her job or responsibility).
4. I desire to spend time with my teen and enjoy being together.
5. My teen is comfortable coming to me when he or she is experiencing joy, satisfaction, guilt, shame, sadness, or a host of other emotions.
6. My teen frequently talks with me and enjoys being with me. I usually listen without preaching, judging, or criticizing. I listen to my teen with the intent to just listen. Even when I don't understand, relate to, or like what my teen is saying, I listen.
7. I understand my teen's temperament, talents, and love language. I let my teen know about his or her unique qualities, gifts, and talents I admire.
8. I know what my teen is capable of achieving, and I help my teen set goals based on what is appropriate for him or her as a unique individual.

❖ Full spoke: I believe seven or eight of the numbered factors are true.

❖ 3/4 spoke: I believe five or six of the numbered factors are true.

❖ 1/2 spoke: I believe three or four of the numbered factors are true.

❖ 1/4 spoke: I believe one or two of the numbered factors are true.

❖ No spoke: None of the numbered factors apply to me and my teen.

Researchers call these two vertical spokes the "parental warmth" or "parental receptiveness" spokes. They deal with your expression of verbal and physical affection toward your teen, as well as your praise and acceptance. Low parental warmth (criticism, disapproval, and rejection of the teen) has been associated with a number of negative health factors and behaviors in teens. In contrast, high warmth has been linked to highly healthy teens.

Now we'll turn from the vertical spokes of the emotional health wheel to its horizontal spokes.

Media/Learning

To come up with the measurement for this left-hand spoke, add the following two factors together.

The first is your teen's exposure to media. One could make the argument that today's teens are overstimulated, and I wouldn't issue a peep of protest. More often than not, too much media in teens' lives—video games, computer games, music DVDs, and way too much television—assaults their senses, negatively affects their minds, and is detrimental to their emotions and body. Many media providers are trying to influence our teens in ways that most parents consider highly unhealthy. Highly healthy parents know how to set limits when it comes to media. Where does your teen line up?

❖ 1/2 spoke: Our home is TV free or my teen watches one hour or less a day, and the computer/Internet is only used in a public area of our home and for educational purposes. If my teen watches TV, I routinely monitor what he or she watches. I monitor what my teen does on the Internet. I put restrictions on the music CDs my teen buys.

❖ 1/4 spoke: My teen is routinely exposed to two hours or less a day of media (television, videos, video games, and computer activities). Also, I sometimes monitor what my teen watches on TV and does on the Internet, and I sometimes put restrictions on the music CDs my teen buys.

❖ No spoke: My teen is routinely exposed to two to four or more hours a day of media, or I never monitor what my teen watches on TV and does on the Internet, and I never put restrictions on the music CDs my teen buys.

❖ Subtract up to 1/4 spoke if your teen has a TV in his or her bedroom or unfettered Internet access in the bedroom.

The second half of this left-hand spoke is your teen's enjoyment of learning and mental activity. Research shows that the brain, like a muscle, must be exercised in order to remain highly healthy. Just as physical activity helps a teen's physiological structure stay healthy, his or her brain benefits from stimulating mental activity—from continuous, active learning. In addition, activities such as reading, doing crossword puzzles, and even playing board games with family members have been linked with sharper minds throughout life. So how much does your teen like to learn?

❖ 1/2 spoke: My teen shows a moderate to high level of enjoyment for mental activities such as reading, ongoing education and learning, challenging mental tasks, good conversation, or board games with the family.

❖ 1/4 spoke: My teen shows little enjoyment for mental activities and learning.

❖ No spoke: My teen shows almost no enjoyment for mental activities and learning.

Boundaries

Teaching a teen to reduce the media he or she is exposed to and setting appropriate expectations and limits compose what researchers call "parental demandingness." When balanced with parental warmth (the love spokes), a teen is more likely to be highly healthy. Too much of one or too little of the other leads to reduced levels of health.

"Parental demandingness" (discipline, expectations, and coaching) is the extent to which a teen's parents expect responsible behavior from their teen and maintain what the researchers call a "hands-on attitude" with their teen. This includes consistently setting and enforcing rules or limits on your teen. Rules for teens, however, must be clear, reasonable, developmentally appropriate, fair and just, mutually agreed upon, and flexible—emphasizing what to do rather than just what not to do.

Measure this spoke based on how many of the following boundaries you consistently impose:

1. I routinely know where my teen is after school and on weekends.
2. I expect to be and am told the truth by my teen about where they are really going.
3. I am aware of my teen's academic performance and visit with his or her teachers from time to time.
4. I impose and enforce a curfew.
5. I make it crystal clear that I would be extremely upset if my teen smoked tobacco or marijuana or used any illicit drugs.
6. I make it crystal clear that I expect intimate sexual activity to be reserved for marriage.
7. I eat dinner with my teen at least five times a week.
8. I assign my teen regular chores.
9. I turn off the TV during dinner and rarely eat in front of the TV.
10. There is an adult present whenever my teen returns from school.

- ❖ Full spoke: Nine or ten of these factors are true for our family.
- ❖ 3/4 spoke: Seven or eight of these factors are true for our family.
- ❖ 1/2 spoke: Five or six of these factors are true for our family.
- ❖ 1/4 spoke: Three or four of these factors are true for our family.
- ❖ No spoke: Zero, one, or two of these factors are true for our family.

RELATIONAL WHEEL

Hub = trust in and nurturing healthy relationships with others and self
Vertical Spokes = relationship with parents and family relationships
Horizontal Spokes = connectedness and performance in school/extracurricular activities

Relationship with Parents

Of all the characteristics of highly healthy parents, other than loving your children unconditionally, the most important is the quantity of time you sacrificially give to your teen. Quality time occurs *only* within quantity time—period and end of discussion.

Your relationship with your teen is critical to his or her self-concept and ability to develop and maintain healthy relationships. Therefore, a critical measure of your relationship is the amount of time you spend with your teen. Use these factors to mark the top spoke of this wheel:

- ❖ Full spoke: Both my spouse and I spend more than thirty minutes each day with our teen.
- ❖ 3/4 spoke: Either my spouse or I spend more than thirty minutes each day with our teen; the other spends between two and three hours each week with our teen.
- ❖ 1/2 spoke: Both my spouse and I spend between two and three hours each week with our teen.
- ❖ 1/4 spoke: Both my spouse and I spend some time but less than two hours weekly with our teen.
- ❖ No spoke: Neither my spouse nor I spend any significant time with our teen.

Family Relationships

The relationship between a teen's parents, as I'll show you later, is a critical factor in the life of a highly healthy teen. What is the quality of family relationships around your teen? Use these factors to mark the bottom spoke of this wheel:

For married, biological parents who live together

- ❖ Full spoke: My spouse and I have a great marriage.
- ❖ 3/4 spoke: My spouse and I have a moderately good marriage.
- ❖ 1/2 spoke: My spouse and I have a marriage fair in quality.
- ❖ 1/4 spoke: My spouse and I have a marriage of poor quality.

For married parents of adopted children who live together

- ❖ 3/4 spoke: My spouse and I have a great marriage.
- ❖ 1/2 spoke: My spouse and I have a moderately good marriage.
- ❖ 1/4 spoke: My spouse and I have a marriage fair in quality.
- ❖ No spoke: My spouse and I have a marriage of poor quality.

For single parents

- ❖ Full spoke: I spend more than thirty minutes each day with my teen. I also involve positive, significant role models of the opposite gender (of the single parent) in my teen's life three hours or more each week.

❖ 3/4 spoke: I spend more than thirty minutes each day with my teen. I also involve positive, significant role models of the opposite gender (of the single parent) in my teen's life at least one hour each week.

❖ 1/2 spoke: I spend at least thirty minutes each day with my teen. I have not yet provided positive, significant role models of the opposite gender (of the single parent) for my teen.

❖ 1/4 spoke: I spend less than thirty minutes each day with my teen. I have not yet provided positive, significant role models of the opposite gender (of the single parent) for my teen.

❖ No spoke: I spend less than two hours each week with my teen. I have not yet provided positive, significant role models of the opposite gender (of the single parent) for my teen.

For parents in blended families

❖ Full spoke: My relationship with my spouse and my stepchildren is great.

❖ 1/2 spoke: My relationship with my spouse and my stepchildren is only moderately good.

❖ 1/4 spoke: My relationship with my spouse and my stepchildren is fair to poor.

❖ No spoke: My teen and I are in a blended family, but I am not married.

Now we'll take into account the horizontal spokes of the relational wheel.

Connectedness

A teen's connectedness to his or her parents and friends is foundational to his or her relational as well as emotional health (since relational and emotional health are intricately interwoven). Connectedness in the parent-teen relationship begins with affirmation, blameless (unconditional) love, and boundaries, which we've already measured as part of the emotional wheel. For relational health, we must realize teens with healthy levels of connectedness not only have strong relationships with good friends; they also exhibit a willingness to interact constructively with others, a can-do attitude, a willingness to tackle new adventures, a sense of optimism, and an ability to make friends comfortably.

Add the following two factors to come up with the measurement of the left-hand spoke:

The connectedness my teen has with his or her friends

- ❖ 1/2 spoke: My teen has terrific relationships with great friends.
- ❖ 1/4 spoke: My teen has fair to moderately good relationships with his or her friends.
- ❖ No spoke: My teen either has poor, negative relationships with his or her friends, or my teen has no friends, or my teen runs with a bad crowd or has friends who are not highly healthy.

My teen's attitudes

1. My teen displays a can-do attitude.
2. My teen displays a willingness to tackle new adventures.
3. My teen displays a sense of optimism.
4. My teen displays an ability to make friends comfortably.

- ❖ 1/2 spoke: My teen displays four of the numbered factors above.
- ❖ 1/4 spoke: My teen displays two or three of the numbered factors above.
- ❖ No spoke: My teen displays zero or one of the above.

Performance in School/Extracurricular Activities

Rate this spoke by the meaningfulness of your teen's work—how he or she is doing in school. Given individual talents, how much is he or she achieving? How is your teen doing in extracurricular activities? Has he or she found at least one healthy activity—an after-school job, a club activity or a sport, a church activity—that gives him or her satisfaction? For this spoke I want you to add the "Performance in School" and "Extracurricular Activities" scores together.

Performance in school

Given my teen's gifts, temperament, and talents—

- ❖ 1/2 spoke: My teen is performing as competently as he or she can.
- ❖ 1/4 spoke: My teen is performing with some competence but not as competently as he or she can.
- ❖ No spoke: My teen isn't performing nearly as competently as he or she can.

Extracurricular activities

- ❖ 1/2 spoke: My teen has found at least one healthy activity—an after-school job, a club activity or a sport, or a church activity—that gives him or her satisfaction.
- ❖ 1/4 spoke: My teen has not found a single healthy activity—an after-school job, a club activity or a sport, or a church activity—that gives him or her satisfaction.
- ❖ No spoke: My teen is involved only in unhealthy activities.

SPIRITUAL WHEEL

Hub = trust in and nurturing a healthy relationship with God
Vertical Spokes = personal relationship with God and prayer
Horizontal Spokes = spiritual instruction and spiritual activity

Personal Relationship with God

I define true, positive spirituality in terms of a personal relationship with God resulting in the visible fruit of the Spirit as listed in Galatians 5:22: love, joy, peace, patience, kindness, goodness, faithfulness, gentleness, and self-control. The greater the depth of a teen's spiritual health, the more likely he or she is to be physically, emotionally, and relationally healthy.

Does your teen have a personal relationship with God that changes him or her from the inside out? Use these factors to mark the top spoke of this wheel:

- ❖ Full spoke: My teen believes in God and shows evidence of a close relationship with him because the internal changes he or she is experiencing yield a great deal of love, joy, peace, patience, kindness, goodness, faithfulness, gentleness, and self-control.
- ❖ 3/4 spoke: My teen believes in God and shows evidence of a reasonably good relationship with him because the internal changes he or she is experiencing yield a reasonably high level of love, joy, peace, patience, kindness, goodness, faithfulness, gentleness, and self-control.
- ❖ 1/2 spoke: My teen believes in God and shows evidence of a moderate relationship with him because the internal changes he's experiencing yield a moderate level of love, joy, peace, patience, kindness, goodness, faithfulness, gentleness, and self-control.

❖ 1/4 spoke: My teen believes in God but shows almost no evidence of a personal relationship with him.
❖ No spoke: My teen does not believe in God.

Prayer

In its simplest form, prayer is an intimate conversation between you and your Creator. Prayer can occur anywhere and anytime. Prayer doesn't require a particular place or position. It can be as simple as thanking God for the good things that happen each day or as complex as a long weekend at a prayer conference.

Prayer is a private endeavor for most folks, so you may have to gently ask your teen how his or her prayer life is going. This might best be done in the context of sharing with your teen your own prayer challenges.

So how often does your teen pray? Use these factors to mark the bottom spoke:

❖ Full spoke: My teen prays every day.
❖ 3/4 spoke: My teen prays a few days each week.
❖ 1/2 spoke: My teen prays only a few times each month.
❖ 1/4 spoke: My child prays only on special holidays or before family meals.
❖ No spoke: My teen never or rarely prays.

Spiritual Instruction

During childhood the foundation for spiritual health is laid most fruitfully by means of the actions of the parents. Spiritual values are more effectively caught than taught. A great deal of what a child is taught through spiritual instruction, however, will last a lifetime. Family Bible reading times, Sunday school classes, confirmation classes, church youth group meetings, church camp activities, and the like all play a role. Be sure to add the "daily or weekly" and the "annual" scores together before recording your total "Spiritual Instruction" results on the left-hand spoke:

Daily or Weekly: Does your teen regularly receive adequate religious instruction?

❖ 1/2 spoke: My teen participates in two or more activities each week, such as attending a faith community; joining in our family's Bible reading; and attending Sunday school classes, confirmation classes, or church youth group meetings.

❖ 1/4 spoke: My teen participates in two or more activities each month, such as attending a faith community; joining in our family's Bible reading; and attending Sunday school classes, confirmation classes, or church youth group meetings each month.

❖ No spoke: My teen participates in few or no religious instruction opportunities.

Annual: Does your teen receive adequate annual opportunities for religious instruction?

❖ 1/2 spoke: My teen participates in two of the following (or similar) activities each year: church camp, vacation Bible school, spiritual retreat, mission trip, or church play.

❖ 1/4 spoke: My teen participates in one of the following (or similar) activities each year: church camp, vacation Bible school, spiritual retreat, mission trip, or church play.

❖ No spoke: My child participates in no annual religious instruction opportunities.

Spiritual Activity

For up to half of this spoke, evaluate your teen's involvement in a faith community; the other half focuses on giving to the community in general. Add the "Involvement" and the "Giving" scores together before recording your total "Spiritual Activity" results on the right-hand spoke:

Involvement: Is your teen actively involved in a faith community in which he or she finds meaningful companionship and camaraderie?

❖ 1/2 spoke: My teen is involved at least weekly in a healthy, positive spiritual community in which he or she receives supportive guidance.

❖ 1/4 spoke: My teen is involved less than weekly but at least monthly in a healthy, positive spiritual community in which he or she receives supportive guidance.

❖ No spoke: My teen is not involved in a spiritual community at all, or our spiritual community is unhealthy.

*Giving: Does your teen give of his or her own resources
to others in his or her neighborhood or community?*

- ❖ 1/2 spoke: My teen gives away time, treasure (money), or talent at
  least monthly by participating in at least one of the following (or similar) activities: volunteering at a soup kitchen, helping a neighbor,
  cleaning up along a roadside, or giving money to a church or charity.
- ❖ 1/4 spoke: My teen gives away time, treasure, or talent once each year
  by participating in at least one of the following (or similar) activities:
  volunteering at a soup kitchen, helping a neighbor, cleaning up along
  a roadside, or giving money to a church or charity.
- ❖ No spoke: My teen rarely, if ever, gives away time, treasure, or talent
  in service to others.

THE WHOLE PICTURE

Now that you've marked the estimated length of the spokes on your teen's
four wheels of health, complete the picture by drawing a wheel from the end
of each spoke. Take a look. Are your teen's wheels round, or are they flat in
spots? Are they approximately the same diameter, or is one much smaller than
the others? If your teen has any severely wobbly wheels, he or she is less than
highly healthy. Could he or she make it out of the driveway on a set of wheels
like you see in the chart on the following page from a high school freshman I
knew well?

Now is the time to begin lengthening the short spokes of your teen's
wheels of health. Reading this book will equip you to do just that. If you take
these principles to heart and apply them, you'll see different spokes lengthen
as you make the decisions a parent who intends to nurture a highly healthy
teen would make.

It's fine at this juncture to identify the flattest wheel or the most broken
spokes. To find the flattest wheel, assign a point count to each spoke of each
wheel. Grade each spoke this way:

- ❖ Full spoke = 4 points
- ❖ 3/4 spoke = 3 points
- ❖ 1/2 spoke = 2 points
- ❖ 1/4 spoke = 1 point
- ❖ No spoke = 0 points

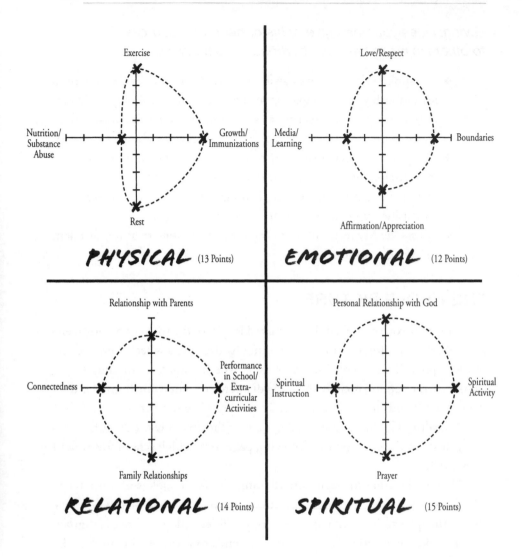

PHYSICAL (13 Points)

EMOTIONAL (12 Points)

RELATIONAL (14 Points)

SPIRITUAL (15 Points)

A perfectly round and fully inflated wheel will have 16 points (4 points for each spoke). In the illustration above, the physical wheel has 13 points, the emotional wheel has 12 points, the relational wheel has 14 points, and the spiritual wheel has 15 points. This boy's spiritual wheel is the healthiest, and his emotional wheel is the least healthy. Since there are three shortened spokes on his emotional wheel, this might be the first one his parents would want to address. If there were equally weakened wheels, I'd recommend parents choose the wheel they think would be the easiest to fix and turn to that area of the book for guidance.

Another option would be to deal with the most broken, or shortest, spokes. Look again at the illustration on page 52, and you'll see that the left-hand spoke on the physical wheel is the shortest of all of this boy's spokes. Another option would be for parents to choose the wheel with the shortest spoke(s). In this case they could choose to begin with the physical wheel. If your teen has more than one spoke that is equally short, choose the one you consider the easiest to address and read the section of the book that deals with that wheel of health. If several are equally short, choose the one you consider the most broken and read the appropriate section. You'll receive some tips for lengthening your teen's spokes on the following pages:

Physical Wheel	chapters 4–7, pages 75–161
Emotional Wheel	chapters 8–10, pages 165–217
Relational Wheel	chapters 11–13, pages 221–65
Spiritual Wheel	chapter 14, pages 269–83

Whether you choose to do something now about your teen's flattened wheel(s) or short spoke(s) or read on and get an overview, this chapter can serve as a reference as you explore ways to equip your teen to live a highly healthy life.

By the way, the illustration on page 52 represents my and Barb's evaluation of our son, Scott, when he was fifteen years old. Barb chose to work with him (and the rest of our family) on the left-hand spoke of the physical wheel, while I volunteered to work with Scott on the horizontal and bottom spokes of his emotional wheel.

Working on these two wheels required much studying and learning on our part. You may have to ask for advice from trusted health care providers and parenting experts. Are you willing to take the necessary actions to help your teens become highly healthy?

It's hard work to nurture highly healthy teens. You may be tempted to stop halfway down the road and let it go at that. Teaching your teens to care for their health will not be simple, just as it's not simple to keep a complex automobile running smoothly. Teens, like cars, require care and upkeep; they need occasional checkups and preventive maintenance to avert problems. The truth is, the human body and mind are hundreds of times more complex than any automobile and thus require even more care and special treatment.

Getting your hands greasy will be worth it. The sacrifice of time and effort will never be wasted. Your effort can and will affect generations to come. Nonetheless, I'd be remiss if I didn't remind you that *not* taking action could cause you great sorrow at some time later in your life.

When Barb and I were raising Katherine and Scott, we tried to implement these principles into their and our lives. We believe Kate and Scott are now highly healthy young adults because of our love, expectations, and efforts. Not only that, Barb and I grew more highly healthy in the process—as individuals and as a married couple.

By the way, if the name Kate rings a bell, it's because she's none other than Katherine Lee Larimore—the Katherine described in chapter 1. And, like her brother, Kate has developed into a highly healthy person, and Barb and I couldn't be more proud of her.

I'll be the first to admit that good parenting does not guarantee good teens. Good parents are vital to highly healthy teens, but I don't want you to think you fully determine the outcome of your teen's decisions. Nevertheless, you are the best chance your teen has of becoming highly healthy.

So are you ready to get started? Let's do so by looking at some beginning steps you can take to nurture and guide your teen into becoming highly healthy.

Chapter 3

WE HAVE IGNITION: PREPARING FOR THE PUBERTY YEARS

The "tweenager" years between eight and twelve can be an awkward time for boys and girls. That's why I liked to liven things up whenever a precocious preteen landed in my examination room. Take Johnny, for example, a gum-smacking eleven-year-old who flipped his ball cap around backward and favored ankle-length cargo pants.

Johnny sat with his mom and tapped out a drumbeat on his legs while I paged through his patient history. Looking up, I cleared my throat to gain his attention. "Have you seen the sex video yet, Johnny?" I casually asked him.

His ears burned after hearing the question. "What sex video?" he wondered aloud, his high-pitched voice rising several octaves.

"Sex video" was my euphemism for *Just Thought You Oughta Know*, a seven-minute, MTV-like production that employs herky-jerky camera work and quick editing cuts to capture the getting-shorter-by-the-minute attention span of today's preadolescents. Between short bursts, hip-looking teens describe the mind-boggling risks of premarital sexual activity—sexually transmitted infections, genital warts, and the HIV virus—to the pounding beat of hip-hop music.

This is in-your-face stuff. In one scene, a teen in dreadlocks holds up a condom package and tears it open. "This is a condom," he says in a deadpan manner, a declarative statement that fits, since this is probably the first time most preteen viewers have seen a prophylactic.

Cut to a new teen guy: "It could protect your penis."

Cut to a teen girl: "It might protect your vagina."

Cut to a teen chorus: "But it won't protect your mind. It can't protect your heart. Just thought you oughta know."

Cue up a rap beat and let it flow: *Just thought you oughta know—Just thought you oughta know.*

It certainly wasn't your mother's sex ed film, showing a horde of spermatozoa swimming crazily to fertilize a solitary egg. What I love about the video is that the message is a 180-degree turn from the "safe sex" teachings that threaten to turn this country into Condom Nation. And that's why I liked showing my sex video to preteens when I was in full-time practice. I have long felt the best time to catch impressionable young minds is *before* the puberty switch is thrown by the pituitary gland.

Check It Out!

▶ You can order your own copy of *Just Thought You Oughta Know* from the Medical Institute for Sexual Health. This intense, award-winning short video features teens talking to teens about the real reasons they can and should delay the onset of sexual activity. For those who are already sexually active, the video encourages them to stop and to begin practicing a healthier lifestyle. After you watch the video with your child, you can pass it along to educators, medical professionals, youth leaders, policy makers, and other parents.

The Medical Institute has released a new video for teens that addresses sex. *Sex Is Not a Game* candidly confronts the dangers of today's casual attitudes about scx and features emotional appearances from teens. This gripping video encourages teens to rethink their risky sexual behavior and save sex for marriage. For more information, contact The Medical Institute, P.O. Box 162306, Austin, TX 78716; call 1-800-892-9484; or visit their website at www.medinstitute.org.

Parental advisory: I always cleared any showing of *Just Thought You Oughta Know* with a parent or guardian. Because of its graphic nature, I encouraged parents to preview it at home or in my clinic before their children viewed it. If I received two thumbs up in the exam room, I directed my nurse, Tish, to roll in a cafeteria cart with a nineteen-inch TV/VCR combo sitting atop. After a few introductory remarks, I'd turn on the video and leave the room to see another patient, but I always returned to make myself available for follow-up questions. It was important to touch base and reaffirm the importance and accuracy of the video's pro-abstinence message. I also used the video to segue to the topic of puberty with Mom or Dad and the preteen.

Puberty (a funny-sounding word pronounced *pyoo*-ber-tee) is a topsy-turvy, potentially explosive time that signals to boys and girls—and their parents—that big changes lie ahead. Young bodies grow very quickly during puberty. Girls start developing curves and go through hairpin mood swings; boys grow muscles and look for the first hair to sprout on the chin.

Puberty still has a way of sneaking up on unsuspecting youngsters—and their parents. I can't tell you the number of mothers who pulled me aside and asked why Sammy shot up four inches over the summer or why Sally's chest size expanded from a 32A to a 34D. Parents who desire to nurture highly healthy teens need to anticipate these tumultuous times so they can stay one step ahead. Their child's young body is growing like the proverbial weed, and the transition from apple-cheeked youngster to full-blown adolescent happens faster than you think!

For that reason I showed *Just Thought You Oughta Know* to audiences as young as eight years old (but I'd only show it to preteens if they were particularly mature or lived in environments where they were exposed to sexual issues very early). And it's why I wrote *Lintball Leo's Not-So-Stupid Questions About Your Body*, a book written for eight- to twelve-year-old boys and their parents about the preteen's changing body and emerging sexual desires. I wanted to reach these impressionable youngsters before their peers did—and, as much as possible, before the media did. I also knew that too many parents were abdicating their role regarding "The Talk," which means their children were learning about sex from the media they encountered, the conversations they had in the neighborhood, and the values-neutral curriculum they were exposed to in school.

IT'S MORE THAN ONE TALK

Parents who wait until their children are twelve or thirteen to have The Talk have waited way too long these days. The time to start talking to your child about sex and the differences between males and females is three or four years of age. You start slowly with little "talks"—not *The* Talk—and you speak in age-appropriate terms. I tried to do that with my children, and I felt my series of little talks over the years adequately prepared my children, Kate and Scott, for their entry into puberty and adolescence.

While I never planned these discussions, I was prepared for them, and I'd urge you to be prepared to take advantage of the spontaneous opportunities that are sure to come your way. When Scott was six or seven years old, he begged me to take him for a ride in my truck. I found an old country road and let him sit on my lap. He eagerly slapped his hands on the steering wheel in the ten and two o'clock position and steered while I worked the accelerator and brakes with my right foot. He loved driving that old truck down that dusty farm road.

Afterward, we stopped for ice cream, and while we licked Rocky Road cones, I eyeballed my son. "Scott, you're really growing," I commented. "Let me see that bicep of yours."

Scott rolled back his T-shirt and struck a Popeye pose, flexing his right bicep but not impressed by the tiny hill that registered on his upper arm. "Daddy, it's not very big."

Lesson time. "It will be, Scott, because your body will begin to change from a boy to a man very soon. Your hormones will do this for you, and when it starts happening, you're going to build big, strong muscles. Believe me, it's coming."

Scott nodded while he took another lick. We were soon talking about something else, but those few sentences were another row of bricks in our foundation of communication. I added another row one time when Barb sat on my lap on the family couch one evening. I felt it was important for the kids to see me hugging Barb and holding her hand as much as possible—and at no particularly special time.

Scott tried to wedge between us. Then, as children sometimes do, he got silly and tried to separate my hand from Barb's.

"How come you're doing that?" I asked, not at all perturbed. I was just wondering what he was up to.

"I want to hold your hand," he said.

"I want to hold your hand too, but nothing comes between me and Mom. Here, you can hold this hand," I said, reaching out with my left, "but this is Mom's hand."

Lesson time. I sensed this was another moment to teach my son something about intimacy. "Right now, God is preparing a wonderful young lady for you, Scott, someone who will be your wife. And you won't want anyone to come between you and her, will you?"

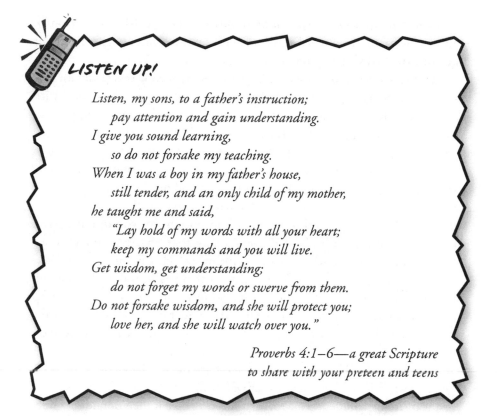

LISTEN UP!

Listen, my sons, to a father's instruction;
    pay attention and gain understanding.
I give you sound learning,
    so do not forsake my teaching.
When I was a boy in my father's house,
    still tender, and an only child of my mother,
he taught me and said,
    "Lay hold of my words with all your heart;
    keep my commands and you will live.
Get wisdom, get understanding;
    do not forget my words or swerve from them.
Do not forsake wisdom, and she will protect you;
    love her, and she will watch over you."

Proverbs 4:1–6—a great Scripture
to share with your preteen and teens

Nevertheless, as your child approaches puberty, you will have to shift gears from talking about sex in general to giving more specific briefings on his or her own sexuality. Whether you make this a separate discussion or include it as part of a more extensive explanation of what lies ahead during the adolescent years, you will want your child to be ready for the physical changes that are about to take place.

For example, girls need to know about breast development, new hair growth, and the reproductive cycle. The first menstrual period should be viewed in a positive light, as a passage into adulthood rather than as a burden or a "curse of women." I would encourage parents to honor this very special occasion by taking their daughter to dinner at a nice restaurant or presenting her with a special gift. This event usually marks the final stage of pubertal development.

Similarly, boys should be aware that changes are on the horizon, such as deepening of the voice, enlarging of the genitals, and new hair growth. They should also know about the likelihood of having unexpected erections and the unanticipated emission of seminal fluid during the night (the "wet dream"), and that neither is a sign of disease or moral failure. Both are gifts from our Creator and part of his perfect design.

Parents will need to talk with their children about the increasing interest they'll be showing in the other gender and how their preteens can deal with the attention they'll receive. It's an important time to review specific guidelines and perhaps share a little street wisdom about relationships and physical contact, all the while reinforcing the importance of saving sex for marriage.

Often these discussions may leave your preteen wondering if you've gone overboard in broaching this subject. Scott once told me, "Dad, I'm not going to jump into bed with any girls, okay? What's the big deal?"

I smiled when he said this. "Scott, it's important for you to understand that we're *all* designed by God in such a way that physical contact, once started, naturally progresses to increasing intimacy." He gave me a funny look, so I explained myself further. "Sex is like a car that begins rolling down a hill. At first, it doesn't seem like you're going so fast, but then things speed up quickly. The farther you get down the hill, the harder it is to stop. It's the same way with sex. Since the right time to have sex is when you're married, you don't want the car to roll very far before the wedding night."

Scott understood my analogy. We even shared a great laugh during his college years when he told me that his car was "still in the garage."

I wanted my children to have a clear notion of what their boundaries were well before they began socializing with the other gender. I wanted my children's childhood and adolescence to be a time for Barb and me to communicate essential points about sex that went far beyond the technical aspects. As a parent, you'll have the privilege and responsibility of emphasizing the wonderful news about sexuality. God designed sex to bring new life into existence, to generate a powerful bond between a husband and wife, and to give a married man and woman an intensely pleasurable experience together. It is a wonderful, extraordinary, and powerful gift that deserves to be treated with great and abiding respect. In the context of a permanent and public commitment, making love should be savored, explored, and nurtured without guilt or fear of serious consequences. When done at the wrong time or with the wrong person, however, sex can bring disappointment, disease, and a derailed life plan.

WHEN THEY'RE READY TO HEAR MORE

As children feel comfortable with various topics, they'll ask the darndest questions, so be ready for the unexpected. Kate must have been about ten years old as we sat at Denny's slurping a milkshake. Out of nowhere, she blurted out, "Dad, what was your wedding night like?"

I nearly choked on my chocolate shake, but I managed to keep my wits. My first order of business was to find out what she was really asking. "What do you mean, Sweetie? Are you referring to where we stayed?"

"No. I was wondering what it was like to be with Mommy *that* night."

I took another deep gulp and then smiled. I was *so* honored that my daughter felt comfortable enough with her dad to ask an honest question. Somehow, I sensed this would be a *very* important moment in our relationship. Mustering an answer I hoped would be appropriate for her age, I said, "It was one of the most amazing nights of our life. We had never been with each other in a bed before. We had never hugged that way, and we had saved ourselves for that night, so it was a night of warmth and talking and touching. That was the night that began our whole marriage."

At ten years of age, that's all Kate needed to hear, but I knew the next time she asked, she'd be ready to hear more. That's why I'm hoping you're reading this book *before* your children get too far into adolescence, but if you haven't, don't sweat it. My goal is to help you nurture highly healthy teens as the full effects of puberty present themselves in your children.

I counsel parents of young teens to stay one step ahead of their children because they are being exposed to sexual discussions at a very young age. Not long ago I was interviewed by the female editor of *CBA Marketplace* on the topic of masturbation for eight- to twelve-year-old boys—a topic I cover in my *Lintball Leo* book for young boys. As we talked about this controversial topic, she told me about raising her fifteen-year-old boy in urban Chicago. "Let me ask you a question about your boy," I said. "Imagine back, seven years ago, when he was eight years old. Would you have wanted to read a book to him that discussed masturbation?"

She paused a second before saying, "Well, we actually talked to him about sex when he was seven years old, but we were two years too late."

Two years? She had to be kidding!

She wasn't. She shrugged her shoulders, signaling that the gritty streets of the Windy City were different from the cul-de-sacs of suburban America. But these days, they're not too much different, thanks to the popular culture as expressed in movies, music, and TV shows. My point is that if you're wondering about when to have The Talk with your preteen or young teen, you're probably too late.

So then, right about now, you may be saying to yourself, *Wait a minute, Dr. Walt. My son is thirteen, and we've barely talked about sex and puberty. What can we do? How can I make up for lost time?*

Answer: Do something about it. If you've been tardy in having The Talk, you need to set the right tone by adopting what I call "the philosophy of apology." Begin by taking your son or daughter to a restaurant. If I were sitting in your seat, here's what I would say:

> Patrick, one of my responsibilities as a parent is to teach you. The Bible says I should teach you day and night, sitting down and standing up. In the next few years, you'll have to make critical decisions that affect your life—decisions about your hobbies, your talents, your career. These are areas where God gives me the responsibility to help prepare you for the future. I hope I've done a good job for you so far.
>
> There is one area, however, where I've failed to do a good job teaching you, and that's the area of sex and intimacy and purity. I want to apologize for this oversight. I goofed, and I hope you'll forgive me.

And away you go. I recommend, if you have a two-parent household, that the father takes the lead in speaking to the son and the mother in speaking to the daughter. Down the road both the father and the mother should participate in these discussions.

If you're talking to a boy who's still on the cusp of adolescence, I'd say something like this:

> Johnny, during the next few years some exciting things will happen that will take you from being a boy to becoming a man. You'll start growing hair around your penis and hair under your arms. Your body will begin producing two things: testosterone and sperm. The testosterone will cause your body to grow, and you'll develop muscles and great strength. The sperm is the body's way of preparing you to become a father. Your testicles produce sperm, and when you make love to your wife, the sperm can fertilize her egg, and then a baby begins growing in her womb.
>
> We can talk more about how all that happens next time, but for now, I want you to know you can ask any question, and no question is too dumb. If I don't know the answer, I'll be sure to get the information for you.

That'll get the discussion ball rolling. Now for you moms, here's what you can say to your daughter:

> Megan, during the next few years some exciting things will happen that will take you from being a girl to becoming a woman. You'll

start having periods, and that's an exciting development because that means you can become a mother. When you make love to your husband, his sperm can fertilize your egg, and then a baby begins growing in your womb.

We can talk more about how all that happens next time, but for now, I want you to know you can ask any question, and no question is too dumb. If I don't know the answer, I'll be sure to get the information for you.

This is the time to call in resources—especially those that have a Christian perspective. Your church library or local Christian bookstore should have books and videos that teach adolescents about sex from a Christian perspective. You can watch those videos together and leaf through the books with your preteens and teens.

Check It Out! ⏪ ▶ ⏸ ⏹ ⏩

▶ An excellent book filled with practical, specific tips on discussing body changes and sexuality with prepubescent and early adolescent children is *A Chicken's Guide to Talking Turkey with Your Kids about Sex* by Dr. Kevin Leman and Kathy Flores Bell.

When I was in practice, we had an extensive patient education library with resources that covered almost any problem a parent would encounter. Your family doctor may offer a similar library, but be careful. His resources may adopt a secular perspective—the material may have a "they're going to do it anyway, so you might as well make sure they're protected" worldview.

It's important for you, the parent, to filter out this "safe sex" ideology. It's a point of view that permeates the public school system, which is why you should be reluctant to turn over your children's sex education to the public schools. All my life I've worked in a field that stresses prevention, but the public school sex ed curriculum turns that philosophy on its head.

Teachers don't say, "Well, we know you're going to drink and drive, so we'll teach you how to drink and drive slowly." That's absurd! They say, "Don't drink and drive. It's dangerous for you, and it can kill innocent people." Nor do teachers say, "Well, we know some of you will do drugs, so we'll show you which drugs not to mix so you'll be safer." That's ridiculous! They say, "Don't do drugs. You'll mess up your mind and your life if you do."

But when it comes to sexual conduct, the public school system often chickens out. It's important for you to be your children's sex education coach during their adolescent years. Remember, if they don't hear it from you, some other source of information will fill that vacuum. As they grow up and gain independence, they will start calling their own plays away from your home-field advantage, so to speak. There isn't anything more important in the next few years than being available to teach them about puberty, about adolescence, about sex, and about relationships with the other gender.

Since it's always a good idea to know what you're talking about, now would be a good time to review what happens to your children's bodies during puberty.

ROAD MAP TO GROWTH

Puberty is the time when children begin to develop physically, emotionally, relationally, and spiritually into young men and women. It starts between the ages of eight and thirteen in girls (the average age is ten) and ten and fifteen in boys (the average age is twelve), but I've seen the average age of puberty drop considerably in my lifetime—perhaps by a year or two. I've evaluated girls as young as six years old for a phenomenon known as "precocious puberty," where the signs of puberty appear before age seven or eight in girls and age nine in boys. Precocious puberty is four to eight times more common in girls than in boys, but it occurs only in one out of every 5,000 to 10,000 U.S. children.

Those who study why these things happen are scratching their heads. Some see the expanding number of obese children as a contributing factor; others say that the higher intake of dairy products containing growth hormones or estrogen may contribute to early puberty. The jury is still out on why children are entering puberty earlier, but the fact is, many of them are. Sometimes medical problems can stimulate precocious puberty, so it's always important that a pediatric endocrinologist evaluate a youngster going through puberty at a young age. Over 85 percent of the time, however, there is no medical problem whatsoever.

Whether puberty starts early, late, or right on time, nothing happens to a young person's body until the brain, acting like a military commander, issues the command for the body to release a special hormone called gonadotropin-releasing hormone, or GnRH in medicalspeak. GnRH travels through the bloodstream and eventually reaches the pituitary gland, a small gland inside the skull and near the bottom of the brain.

The GnRH causes the pituitary gland to perk up and issue its own set of commands, barking orders for two more puberty-causing hormones (gonadotropins) to get marching: luteinizing hormone (LH) and follicle-stimulating hormone (FSH). When these battalions of hormones march into the bloodstream, bodily changes happen rapidly.

Many parents think that boys and girls receive different growth-producing hormones, since the outcomes (sperm and muscles for him and menstruation and breasts for her) are so different, but that's not true. The fact is, these LH and FSH hormones go to work on different parts of the body. For boys, the hormones travel through the bloodstream to the testicles, where they inform the testes to begin making both testosterone and sperm. Testosterone is the vroom-vroom hormone that causes most of the changes to a guy's body during puberty. Muscles grow, hair sprouts around the genitals, and young singers are asked to leave the Vienna Boys Choir.

FH and LSH have different targets inside girls' bodies—the ovaries. These hormones inform the ovaries to start producing estrogen and progesterone on the double, preparing the body to begin the menstrual cycle and release an egg each month. The first manifestation is a budding of the breasts somewhere between the ages of ten and eleven, on average. Pubic hair appears about a year later, followed by a growth spurt.

Menstruation begins two or three years later, which means that most girls are around twelve- to twelve-and-a-half-years-old when they experience their first period. My good friend Tom Fitch, M.D., who is a superb pediatrician, told me, "I don't know where I first read this, but over the past thirty years I've found it to be true in my practice. I tell girls that after their first period, they can expect another two to four inches of height. I say it's a ballpark estimate, but I haven't had many less than two inches or more than four inches, and it's always been more on the high rather than on the low side."

Both sexes experience rapid growth and weight gain during puberty, but what flusters parents is the way children change rather rapidly from sweet, compliant kids to fire-breathing dragons who ask "Why?" and "How come I have to do that?" a lot more often. They begin to (or at least pretend to) listen more to their peers than to their parents, and Dad and Mom—whom they placed on pedestals during the elementary school years—are about as cool as Ken and Barbie dolls dressed in disco clothes.

This development shell-shocked many parents in my practice because they simply underestimated the impact of the myriad of biochemical changes that occur during puberty. The importance of understanding this glandular upheaval is that it should help you tolerate the physical, emotional, relational, and spiritual reverberations that occur during puberty.

I hate to be the bearer of bad news, but your teens will not be perfectly normal during this time—or entirely rational either. Teens in the midst of wild hormonal gyrations may not interpret their world accurately. They are changing day to day—but there is hope. There is much you can do to ensure that the metamorphosis will result in a beautiful and unique creature—and not a werewolf!

A reminder, though: not only are average teens hormonally challenged; they are socially challenged too. Their greatest anxiety and most deadly dread, even exceeding the fear of death, is the possibility of rejection or humiliation by their friends or peers. Since their sense of worth is dependent on the opinion and acceptance of their peers, their friends will hold an enormous influence over your teens.

THE IMPORTANCE OF REGULAR FAMILY ROUTINES

The hormones and social forces squaring off against your teens are a double whammy. That's why it'll be doubly hard to talk about puberty while they're going through it, but if they haven't heard from you, you're going to have to do it. The good news is that it's never too late. The research is reasonably clear that parents are highly effective, both by the example they set and the words they say—and your words are *much* more effective and influential than your teens let on. I've discovered a veritable mountain of research that supports the idea that parents and family ties are among the most influential factors, if not *the* most important factor, in a child's development and well-being.

My first example comes from a recent "Child Trends Report" on family strength. The research emphasized the importance of family and parents:

❖ Regular family routines (meals, chores, and errands) are linked to a teen's academic achievement and self-esteem.
❖ Teen-parent time together helps motivate education and socialize teens.
❖ High parental involvement during high school increases the likelihood that teens will attend college, vote, and volunteer.
❖ Teens closely supervised by their parents are less likely to engage in early or frequent sexual relations.

❖ Teens who receive communication and praise are less at risk for delinquency and alcohol and drug use.

❖ Teens whose parents demonstrate warm support and simultaneously high demands for appropriate behavior tend to be content, self-reliant, and self-controlled.

The parents' role of instilling values in teens remains one of the most influential aspects of parenting. Many parents I speak to seem surprised to learn that their teens still care about their parents' approval.

A study carried out by the Institute for Youth Development (IYD) asked teens what factor most affected their decision about whether to have sex. Thirty-nine percent answered that the morals, values, or religious beliefs taught to them by their parents influenced them the most. The study also reported that hands-on parents raised teens who drank, smoked, and did drugs at much lower rates than the general teen population.

What is a hands-on household? Simply put, it is a home in which parents consistently implemented ten or more of the following twelve actions:

❖ Monitor what their teens watch on TV
❖ Monitor what their teens do on the Internet
❖ Put restrictions on the music CDs their teens buy
❖ Know where their teens are after school and on weekends
❖ Expect to be and are told the truth by their teens about where they are really going
❖ Are very aware of their teens' academic performance
❖ Impose a curfew
❖ Make clear they would be extremely upset if their teen used marijuana
❖ Eat dinner with their teens six or seven times a week
❖ Assign their teen regular chores
❖ Turn off the TV during dinner
❖ Have an adult present when the teen returns from school

Hands-on parents are incredibly important in the lives of teens. A 1996 *Journal of Family Issues* article observed that "family disruption and lack of parental involvement during childhood correlated with an increase in lying, cheating, fighting, and criminal activity among youth."

Hands-on parenting always involves spending lots of time with children. In his article "The Parent Trap," William Mattox Jr. quoted Harvard University child psychiatrist Robert Cole: "The frenzied need of children to have possessions isn't only a function of the ads they see on TV. It's a function of their hunger for what they aren't getting—their parents' time."

When 1,500 schoolchildren were asked, "What do you think makes a happy family?" the most frequent answer was not money, nice houses, cars, or TVs. The most frequent answer was "doing things together" as a family.

YOU'RE PASSING MORE THAN THE POTATOES

Even for hands-on parents, puberty can be a very scary—or at least unsettling—time. I can remember when Kate was entering puberty, and the going was getting tougher for Barb and me. We decided to read a book called *Preparing for Adolescence*, in which well-known child psychologist Dr. James Dobson addressed parents about puberty. The message I remember is that parents needed to know two things: (1) During puberty, the river of adolescence that teens travel down can become very rough and bumpy. That was the bad news. The good news? (2) Eventually the waters will become calm again, and puberty will end. But while these adolescents are on the river, preparation and prayer are key!

It's important for parents to understand that puberty can be a scary time for kids. They'll need you to paddle in the raft with them and help them get through the rapids. What they don't need is for you to stay uninvolved, watching from the shoreline. This sort of commitment will gobble up scads of time because hands-on parents are "time with" parents. I'm talking about driving them to breakfast on Saturday morning, treating them to a Starbucks Mocha Frappuccino after church, and shooting baskets in the driveway before dinner. Stay-at-home moms have a built-in advantage in this department: cars and vans are great places to have communication-building discussions as they're hauling their children to school, soccer practice, and piano lessons.

The key is making the effort to be there for your teens. If you feel you couldn't put in the necessary time up to now, you'll need to start at a slower speed. Fathers, you can't decide, after having read this chapter, to suddenly spend twelve hours next Saturday taking your son to IHOP for waffles, sweeping up leaves with him in the yard, catching the college football game on TV in the afternoon, and taking in a movie with him that night. Most teens can't transition that quickly—especially if you've made the mistake of not investing time in your children when they were younger. Going from twelve minutes a day to twelve hours overloads the circuits. If you haven't been there with them when they were younger, they've undoubtedly developed other support groups and have other resources. Somewhere along the line they may have received a strong message from you that other things were more important, and so they moved on. They didn't want to, but they felt as though they had no choice. Winning them back will take time and patience, and it will involve learning how to speak their love language.

LISTEN UP!

When a child turns 13, you put him in a barrel with only a hole to feed him through. When he turns 16, plug the hole.

Mark Twain, author and humorist

LEARN TO SPEAK THEIR LANGUAGE

I heard about the love languages of teens from author Gary Chapman, who says teens feel loved when

- ❖ parents verbally affirm them;
- ❖ parents give them affectionate touches and close hugs;
- ❖ parents spend quality time with them;
- ❖ parents serve them; and
- ❖ parents give them gifts.

As you may guess, buying nice things for your teens isn't enough and, by itself, can be very harmful. Teens don't need *things* from their parents; they need *their parents*—their unconditional love, their cheerleading, their advice and guidance, their steering and teaching, and, most of all, their time and prayers. As a parent, you need to love your teens by employing all five of these love languages, while also discovering your teens' primary love language.

As my daughter grew older, I realized that my primary love language was hearing words of affirmation, but it was *not* Kate's primary love language. I could give her words of affirmation all day long, and while she appreciated it, those words never communicated love to her in the same way her primary language would have. I learned that Kate's primary love language is affectionate touches and close hugs. Her secondary language is words of affirmation—but her primary language is huddle and cuddle.

Now, while not every teen's primary love language is having someone spend quality time with them, the fact is, *every* teen needs parents to spend quality time with them. It's critical to learn, as I did, that quality time can only occur within quantity time—a concept I learned when I read a book written by Richard Swenson, a family physician. In *Margin*, Dr. Swenson explained how families are being destroyed by parents (and dads particularly) who leave no margin in their schedule for their kids. I read this book just as Kate was approaching adolescence. My typical schedule consisted of morning rounds at the hospital, followed by seeing patients in the office for six hours a day (from 9:00 a.m. to noon and 2:00 p.m. until 5:00 p.m.) and going back to the hospital for evening rounds. This schedule left little margin for me to spend time with my children.

Dr. Swenson's book galvanized me to do something about that. I met with my medical partner, and we agreed to a new working arrangement: On Tuesdays and Thursdays, I'd see patients from 8:00 a.m. until 2:00 p.m. and be home by 3:00 p.m. to meet one of our children at the bus stop. Tuesday afternoons and evenings were for Kate—and for her alone. Thursdays were for Scott. We'd ride bikes. We'd go fishing. We'd go get a milkshake. We'd take long walks and have long talks about anything and everything. Then we'd go home and work on homework together.

LISTEN UP!

Create margin in your life. Margin means establishing parameters that leave you energy at the end of the day, money at the end of the month, and sanity at the end of your child's adolescence. Marginless, on the other hand, is being thirty minutes late for your son's basketball game because you were twenty minutes late getting out of a meeting because you were ten minutes late getting back from lunch.

Richard Swenson, M.D., author of Margin

I had a blast! I got to know and love my kids in ways that could never have happened any other way. I learned firsthand that quality time occurs *only* in the midst of quantity time. Sure, Kate and Scott needed positive affirmation, emotional support, and nurturing from me. But more than that, they needed my time.

Several years later, when Kate was nineteen, I was invited to introduce Dr. Swenson at a medical conference for physicians and their spouses. Kate was at the meeting with me, and when she heard that Dr. Swenson was there, *she* wanted to introduce him. Here's what she said that afternoon:

> Ladies and gentlemen, when I was a little girl, my daddy read a book that Dr. Swenson had written. The book was called *Margin*. In that book, my daddy learned that if he wanted me to be as healthy as I could be, he would have to spend some time with me—a lot of time. He would need to create margin into his schedule and into his world for me. So my daddy took time away from work and spent every Tuesday afternoon and evening with me. He has never given me a more wonderful gift. I will never forget the memories I have from those days.

Then my daughter turned to the author of *Margin* and said, "Dr. Swenson, I want to thank you for teaching my daddy. Because of what he did, I will never be the same."

She then turned back to the audience. "Dr. Swenson is going to teach today on parenting. I encourage you to listen, as my daddy did, so that you can change the life of your kids the way my daddy changed mine."

As Kate sat down to tumultuous applause, I don't mind telling you that both Dick Swenson and I wiped away tears from our eyes.

Parents, hear this loud and clear: highly healthy kids depend on their relationships with their moms *and* their dads. Loving parents who give their kids both love and time give them a greatly increased shot at becoming highly healthy. If your own parents didn't give you this gift, you have a chance to break the cycle with your children. If your kids are grown, then perhaps you can influence the relationship your kids have with your grandkids. It's worth the effort.

Now that you have a better understanding of both the physiological changes teens go through and the importance of investing time in communicating with your teens, let's turn our attention to our teens' physical wheel. For this age group, appearance is a big deal. There's a lot to talk about in the next chapter, and I think you'll find it practical and helpful.

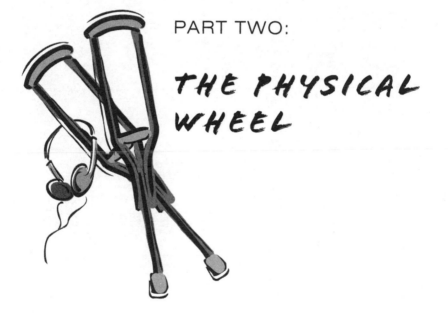

PART TWO:

THE PHYSICAL WHEEL

YOU'RE TWO-THIRDS OF THE WAY THERE

When Kate turned six years old, my father called her on the telephone to wish her a happy birthday. I beamed like any proud dad, and then Kate turned to me. "Pop would like to speak with you," she said as she handed me the phone.

"Congratulations," my father declared.

His comment confused me. "For what, Dad? What did I do?" I asked.

"It's Kate's one-third birthday."

Now I was really confused. "She's six years old, Dad."

"Yes, but one-third of your life with her is over."

One-third? You mean I was one-third of the way raising this little pipsqueak of a girl who favored coloring books and being read to? It didn't seem possible. She was so tiny. But I instantly understood what my father was saying: at eighteen, she's going to leave home, and your child-rearing days will be over.

Let's do a little extrapolation. If you have a twelve-year-old child in the house, your child-rearing days are two-thirds complete. More than halfway home. You're rounding the clubhouse turn, and the finish line is in sight. Just like any horse race, though, the homestretch is the toughest real estate to cover, and there will be times in the next six years that you're sure your little jockey is taking the whip to your flanks.

Blame it on hormones. The river of testosterone and estrogen coursing through your child's veins and arteries produces explosive outbursts and wild mood swings. Young adolescents have a way of changing their countenance from happy to sad, calm to angry, stimulated to depressed—all in the same minute!

Their emotions mimic the ups and downs of a day at Wall Street. When your teens are happy, they can be exceedingly joyful. When they're sad, they can become downhearted, even suicidal. When they're upbeat, they're excited and pumped. When they're angry, they rail against the heavens and slam bedroom doors.

Mood swings are often manifestations of difficulties coping with physical changes. Every time your young adolescents turn around, they seem to hear that timeworn phrase "My, how you've grown!" from well-meaning grandparents and other relatives, along with a pat on the back. That can be exasperating, but it's the attention of their peers that scares them the most. Think about the overweight or obese child who enters adolescence and has to deal with the jeers, the put-downs, and the bullying that overweight kids so often experience. Or think about young girls with budding breasts who aren't certain what to make of the boys' sudden wide-eyed attention as they walk the school halls.

Puberty brings new concerns about body image and appearance. Both girls and boys who never gave much thought to their looks suddenly spend hours primping in front of the bathroom mirror, worrying about a zit on their chin or complaining about being too short, too tall, too fat, or too skinny. Body parts grow at different times and rates; the hands and feet, for example, often grow faster than the arms and legs. Because walking and talking and running and reaching require coordination, young adolescents feel like they're going through life dribbling two basketballs at the same time.

Not only do boys' fast-growing feet look strange; they also *smell* strange, thanks to testosterone. Besides building strong bodies, testosterone affects the glands in the skin. When testosterone seeps into the skin pores, these glands produce a chemical reaction, and the smell isn't reminiscent of cologne. Think *eau de stinky socks*.

The feet reek, and the underarms—well, you don't want to take a sniff there! Parents can help by encouraging the use of deodorants and by washing their tennis shoes every few weeks. Foot powder can do wonders as well.

Ah, the joys of going through puberty! One thing I always emphasize to parents is that puberty will rock their world and their children's. It's a tumultuous time with peaks and valleys, which means parents need to do two things: (1) hang on for the ride of their lives, and (2) know that one day it will end. Whether adolescence ends peacefully and harmoniously or ends in strife and hard feelings depends largely on what you do between the beginning and the end of puberty.

That's why you want to become an expert on teens, learning everything you can about these fascinating and sometime frustrating creatures. You'll need this information so you can employ savvy negotiating skills and find the right balance between giving them independence and squashing their spirits. Barb and I knew we weren't experts when Kate, our oldest, entered puberty, so we sought the advice of other parents who had been down that road. We asked our close friends Bill and Jane Judge if we could call on them when we became overwhelmed. They had raised five children, and since experience is often the best teacher, we figured they'd be great mentors for Barb and me—which turned out to be true, as the following story illustrates.

One of our household traditions was my putting the kids to bed each night I was home. I would supervise putting their pajamas on, brushing their teeth, and reading them a bedtime story. Kate and Scott had their own bedrooms, so I'd put one child to bed first and then the other.

After a bedtime story, we would pray together, and then I'd give the kids a chest rub or a back rub. The next morning, I would wake the kids up with a gentle chest rub while singing a cock-a-doodle-doo song. One morning, when Kate was around ten or eleven years old, I sang my good-morning ditty and rubbed her chest, as per my custom. She smiled and stretched while I rubbed her chest, but then my hand ran across something I hadn't noticed before—speed bumps. *Oh, my goodness!* I freaked out because I was touching her—her . . .

So I quit rubbing her chest in the mornings. Instead, I would walk into the room, sing the cock-a-doodle-doo song, and wish her a good morning. "Time to wake up," I'd say.

I happened to mention this development to Bill Judge. "Bill, you've had five daughters. Did this ever happen to you?" I asked.

"You bet," he responded. "It happens to every dad, so don't worry about it. Your girl is becoming a woman. But did I hear you right? Did you say you stopped rubbing your daughter's chest?"

"Yes. I don't want to touch her inappropriately."

"That's fine, but teens need touch, and if you don't touch her, if you don't hug her, if you don't hold her, she'll seek it from someone else. You can and should touch her. Just find some other place on her body to rub that's entirely appropriate."

What Bill said was a great encouragement to me. That evening, as I was putting Kate to bed, I said, "Have you noticed that I haven't been rubbing your chest in the morning?"

Kate scrunched up her nose. "Yeah, I *have* noticed. How come?"

"Well, you're changing in that area, and as your breasts grow, that's a place that's off-limits to Dad, and it's reserved for your future husband. I still want to give you back rubs and shoulder rubs though."

"That would be great, Dad."

I don't think I would have thought of that without Bill's guidance, and it was just one of many occasions on which I sought his advice. I highly recommend you think of a couple you can use as a sounding board during the teen years. We all need mentors who have experience and insights on their side.

The Bible is filled with examples of mentoring—Eli and Samuel, Elijah and Elisha, Moses and Joshua, Naomi and Ruth, Elizabeth and Mary, Paul and Timothy. Up until a hundred or so years ago, multiple generations of the same family usually lived in the same village or tended the same farm together. Older family members and next of kin were great resources to call on.

Today, living near grandparents is the exception, not the rule. That's why we should seek out mentors we can bounce ideas and situations off. Such arrangements can be formal ("Hey, could you be a mentor in helping me nurture my teens?") or informal (asking your friends a casual question about parenting when something comes up)—whatever you feel comfortable with.

FYI . . .

► *One Swerve Away*

The leading cause of death among American teens is not teen suicide or cancer; it's motor vehicle crashes. Young people between the ages of fifteen and twenty make up 6.7 percent of the total driving population, but they are involved in 14 percent of all car fatalities.

By every statistical measurement, teens are poor drivers. They're four times more likely than older drivers to get into wrecks; more likely to underestimate the dangers of hazardous situations; and more likely to speed, run red lights, make illegal turns, not wear their seat belts, ride with intoxicated drivers, and drive after using alcohol or drugs. That's why insurance companies, who study where their payouts go, slap the highest premiums on teen drivers.

I'm in favor of a graduated license program—something thirty-seven states have enacted in one form or another. Young drivers must complete advanced driver education training, adhere to passenger restrictions (meaning no joyriding with their friends), and observe nighttime driving restrictions. We practiced a modified graduated license program with Scott. We paid for driving lessons from a twenty-five-year veteran of teaching teens to drive, and then Scott had to drive with either me or Barb for months and months before we allowed him to drive alone. When he proved he was responsible, we granted him driving privileges while retaining the right to approve whom he drove with and where.

My collaborative writer Mike Yorkey shares his story about how he and his wife, Nicole, handled teen driving in their household:

> It's become a rite of passage out here in Southern California: on your teen's sixteenth birthday, you pull Missy out of school so she can take her driver's test at the nearby DMV. If all goes well, she'll have a temporary license in her hands by noon—and plenty of time to share the good news with her squealing friends back at school. No wonder why they call it the "Sweet Sixteen" birthday.
>
> I can understand the urgency behind sixteenth-birthday driving exams. For teens, the keys to a car represent freedom of movement, the chance to escape the parental leash of relying on Mom and Dad for wheels. Family experts say a driver's license is a tangible sign that the child is growing up and ready to accept the responsibility of operating a motor vehicle.
>
> So consider the pressure my wife, Nicole, and I felt as Andrea, our oldest child, steadily moved toward her sixteenth birthday. All her school friends had shiny new licenses in their wallets and shiny new cars in the school parking lot, but it was looking as though we couldn't afford either. I had recently left a job where I didn't get paid for nearly six months (a long story), and we were struggling to keep the family's financial ship afloat. To bring in some cash, I was working at home on book projects and magazine articles. It was a time to hunker down and ride out the stormy financial waters. Any frivolous

expenses were tossed overboard, and that included any dreams Andrea might have had about getting her own car.

In addition, we were concerned about turning Andrea loose on the traffic-choked streets of Southern California. We had heard the stories about her classmates' driving escapades: the girl who rolled her father's prized Mercedes, the boy who drove the family SUV into San Elijo lagoon, and so on. Thankfully, none of Andrea's friends were hurt, but the high number of teen accidents caused us to wonder if the "freedom" of driving a car was worth the price.

When we informed Andrea that we didn't have the money to put her on our insurance plan, she was fine with that. I think she knew she wasn't ready to jostle for room on San Diego's fast-paced freeways, and she agreed that the surface streets were an accident waiting to happen. We promised, however, to drive her anywhere she wanted after school or on weekend nights, as long as the trip made sense.

Another reason Andrea went along with our plan is because neither Nicole nor I had gotten our driver's licenses on our sixteenth birthdays. I told Andrea my mother let my six-teenth birthday slide by with nary a peep about getting my driver's license, and it wasn't until I tactfully brought the subject up months later that she reluctantly allowed me to take my driver's test. Nicole grew up in Switzerland, where the magic age is eighteen before you can drive. According to my wife's thinking, if she had to wait until eighteen, then her daughter could too.

So Andrea would have to wait, but she was a great sport about it. For two years, we chauffeured her everywhere until she took her driver's test a few days before her eighteenth birthday. And that two-year delay turned out to be one of the best things to happen to our family. Here's what we serendipitously learned:

1. *Teens can survive just fine without a driver's license at age sixteen.* Hey, we live in car-happy Southern California,

where automotive mobility is a must, but we managed just fine. I think whoever wrote the laws allowing teens to drive at sixteen didn't think through the sociological conditions behind such a directive. Maybe sixteen-year-olds could handle driving the family Model T to the general store seventy-five years ago, but driving a few miles on an uncrowded country road back then is far different from negotiating the merge into four lanes of heavy freeway traffic today. Nicole and I felt Andrea wasn't ready to drive at sixteen because it wasn't right to let her handle all that stressful traffic. Maybe the Swiss know something we don't.

2. *Not having a license didn't cramp Andrea's social calendar at all.* Remember, we told Andrea we'd drive her any-where, anytime. What it meant in actual practice was many Saturday nights driving her to the bowling alley to meet her friends and picking her up at midnight to bring her home (a one-hour round-trip). We picked her up from school, ran her around town for tennis lessons, drove her to her friends' homes, and waited outside the homecoming dance just before the carriage turned into a pumpkin. No complaining on our end.

3. *We got to spend more time with Andrea.* Here's the hidden benefit no one thinks about: we got to spend more time with Andrea during her high school years. Nicole drove her and her brother to school every day. Driving her back and forth to places like the bowling alley guaranteed us more hours to talk and to share her evening. We got to hear about (and meet) her friends. We remained very involved during an important time of her life.

4. *We saved a ton of money.* Did you know that the cost to drive a fairly ordinary new car—a standard-issue Ford Taurus or Nissan Altima—is more than fifty cents per mile? This means a ten-mile trip to the local mall costs five bucks. I'll concede that the cost of driving a well-used car—okay, a beater—would be a bit less, but even at 40 cents per mile, a one-hundred-mile round-trip

drive to a concert would be $40. So at the end of the year, the cost to drive 10,000 miles—plus the cost of gas, oil changes, repairs, new tires, license fees, and insurance (sky-high for teens!)—would be a figure well north of $4,000. Sure, there were costs associated with driving Andrea everywhere she wanted to go, but we could rein in some of those expenses (car insurance, gas fill-ups, and wear and tear on the car).

By the way, our son, Patrick, was willing to wait too. He's sixteen months younger than Andrea, so when he turned sixteen, Andrea still didn't have her license. Our financial situation had eased some but not our concern about teen drivers. So Patrick agreed to wait until the summer before his senior year (when he was seventeen years, three months) to get his driver's license.

No pun intended, but we can say the wait didn't kill him. Based on our experience, we'd urge you not to give in to the "they gotta have their driver's license the day they turn sixteen" philosophy. Waiting until they turn eighteen is probably too long, but age seventeen sounds good.

I know some parents can't wait until their children can drive so they can help with the family carpooling. But if you're looking for less stress, less worry, more money in your pocket, and more time with your children, leave the driving to you—not them!

A BREAKDOWN OF TEENS' GROWTH

Let's revisit the physical changes your teens can expect during puberty. If your children fall into the normal growth range, they can expect to add inches to their frame and weight to their torsos over the next few years. Because you see them each day, you may not notice how fast they're growing unless you're keeping a record of their growth on a basement wall or a bedroom doorjamb.

That's why you need to be aware of what's coming up so you can tell your teens what to expect. Let's break down some of the differences in physical changes between the genders, keeping in mind that girls mature one to two years sooner than boys do.

Where the Boys Are

The physical difference between a young boy and a young man can take a parent's breath away, especially when you consider that today's generation will be one inch taller and weigh about ten pounds more than their fathers. The age of a girl's first period is dropping like an elevator, but guys aren't far behind—they're reaching sexual maturity about nine months earlier than their fathers.

I can't overemphasize the fact that puberty begins at different times and lasts for different periods of time for each boy. The process can begin as early as nine years of age and as late as fourteen years of age. For boys, puberty can last from two to five years. Teen boys who have late onset of puberty face special challenges, especially if they get teased by their peers in PE class. No one likes being called "bald eagle" when his classmates already have a bushel of hair around their penises.

Wise parents will want to give their late blooming sons some extra tender loving care. It's an especially critical time for Dad to be on the scene. Since the acorn doesn't fall too far from the tree, it's possible that Dad was a bald eagle when he was his son's age. If that was true for you, Dad, it's now time to have a private discussion with your son. Share what you are observing and ask open-ended questions. Give your son time to sort through his thoughts and insecurities. Share how you felt at his age and reassure him that God's not done with him—not by a long shot!

Growing Up, Up, and Up

Puberty causes your sons to go through an incredible growth spurt—an average of about four inches of height per year. This compares to the average of 2.3 inches per year in the prepubertal male. I want to reiterate that different parts of your teen's body will grow at different times and rates. His head, hands, and feet are the first body parts to grow. Then the arms and legs grow in length and definition. Finally, the torso, shoulders, and hips catch up by the end of adolescence. No wonder adolescence is an awkward time!

Although boys usually begin their growth spurt one to two years after the girls, they continue to grow for three to four years after most girls have stopped growing. Therefore, boys may not complete their physical growth until they are twenty or twenty-one.

Five Stages of Puberty for Boys

Doctors and developmental experts use the Tanner Classification of development and its five stages to help them better understand puberty:

Stage 1: From birth until about nine to twelve years old—
the average end of this stage is about ten years old

The male hormones begin their activity toward the end of this stage, but there are very few, if any, outward signs of development. The testicles are maturing, and some boys start a period of rapid growth late in this stage. Testicular enlargement is something to look for during puberty. If there is evidence of testicular enlargement before the ninth birthday or no evidence of pubertal changes by the fourteenth birthday, there are reasons for concern, and your child must be evaluated by a doctor.

Stage 2: Usually nine to fifteen years old—
the average end of this stage is twelve to thirteen years old

The testicles and scrotum begin to enlarge, but penis size doesn't increase much. In the early stages of puberty, the scrotal skin can redden, occasionally itch, and change texture. Very little, if any, pubic hair appears at the base of the penis. However, there is an increase in height and a change in body shape.

Stage 3: Usually eleven to sixteen years old—
the average end of this stage is thirteen to fourteen years old

The penis starts to grow in length but not much in width. The testicles and scrotum are still growing. Pubic hair starts to get darker and coarser and spreads toward the legs. Height growth continues, and the shape of the body and face looks more like an adult. The voice begins to deepen and can crack. Some hair grows around the anus.

Stage 4: Usually eleven to seventeen years old—
the average end of this stage is fourteen to fifteen years old

Pubic hair begins to take adult texture, although it covers a smaller area, and the penis widens and grows in length. Then, within a year of the penis starting to grow, most boys will have their first ejaculation, which can occur as a wet dream. For many boys, this can be scary or even worrisome; the same is true for parents (especially moms), who might wonder if this indicates poor morals. Not to worry! These uncontrollable ejaculations are perfectly natural and designed to be part of a boy's growth and development. Involuntary erections are also a frequent occurrence during this time. It takes very little stimulation (visual, mental, or physical) to elicit an erection in a young man—and often the stimulus is not recognized or desired. Facial hair increases on the chin and upper lip. The voice gets deeper, and the skin gets oilier. Acne can appear about the same time as the sprouting of underarm hair.

Stage 5: Usually fourteen to eighteen years old—
the average end of this stage is about sixteen years old

Your teen is nearing his full adult height and physique. Pubic hair and genitals have an adult appearance. Facial hair grows more completely, and shaving may begin now or soon. During the late teens and early twenties, some men grow a bit more and develop more body hair, especially chest hair.

Boys who are slower to develop than their peers often wonder if there's any way they can make the penis grow more quickly, especially if they're reading those ads in the sports pages or in the email spam that promise "penis enhancement." Two things you need to convey to your boys: (1) there is *no* healthy or natural way to increase penis size, and (2) when it comes to sex, size doesn't matter.

Breast Development

Many boys experience the slight growth of one or both breasts during puberty. Yes, you read this right, and I've treated more than a few anxious adolescent boys who had developed small breasts. They usually made an appointment with me because they were being teased in the community shower after PE. Some were sure they were dying or, even worse, turning into girls.

"No, you are not turning into a girl," I'd say on those occasions, and I could see the palpable relief in their faces. "You are not dying. This is not cancer. This is just God's design at work in you."

I'm sure many young boys think God was doodling instead of doing some real designing when it came to puberty. What most people don't know is that gynecomastia (pronounced: *guy-neh-coh-mass-tee-uh*) is very common for boys during puberty—nearly half of all young boys develop a tender nodule right under the nipple. The tender breasts (or breast, since it can occur in only one) may discharge a clear or slightly milky fluid, especially if they are squeezed or manipulated.

Parents sometimes get uptight when their sons develop small breasts, but listen, it's not something to stress over. Nevertheless, if you're concerned about gynecomastia, be sure to have your doctor take a look. He or she can do a brief exam and usually put your and your son's minds at ease. Remember, although it may be embarrassing for you, it's everyday stuff for your doctor. The good news is that a bit of breast growth and tenderness is a temporary condition that goes away over time.

Here are a few tips to help your son get through this time:

❖ Have him wear loose-fitting shirts, which helps make gynecomastia less noticeable and decreases the tenderness.

❖ Urge him to avoid rubbing his breasts because such stimulation can actually increase the growth and the time it will take for the breasts to shrink to normal size.

❖ Remind him that the condition is temporary. Gynecomastia is just another aspect of puberty—the process God designed as a way to turn a young boy into a powerful man of God.

Voice Change

A boy's voice will slowly deepen during puberty, which is a good thing. No longer will he be mistaken for his mom or his sisters on the phone. The process is gradual and almost always results in his voice breaking at times. Don't laugh at him or tease him. This completely normal and natural process occurs in virtually every boy, and you can assure your teen that this is yet another thing that will pass.

Voice changes represent just one of the many changes boys experience and worry about. Even though they may be able to talk about their problems and develop some problem-solving skills, they still need special help and support from their parents. During early adolescence, teens are sensitive to disapproval or criticism. Even well-meant advice from a parent can sound like condemnation, which can trigger anger or defiant responses. Teens often respond to the stress of body changes and voice changes by withdrawing and not communicating, by becoming rebellious, and by emotional outbursts.

What can you do to help your sons? Understand that they need to find constructive ways to deal with stressful situations and body changes. As your teens learn that they can deal with problems, they gain a positive attitude about themselves. Perhaps the most effective way to help them manage these changes is to keep the lines of communication open. Although they may not want your advice, they'll almost always appreciate your attention. Most young adolescents just want someone to hear what they have to say.

Body Hair

Your son's facial hair will normally appear about two years after pubic hair sprouts around the penis. Facial hair first appears at the corners of the upper lip and then spreads to the upper lip. It soon crops up on the upper parts of the cheek, below the bottom lip, and finally the sides of the face and the chin. Simultaneously, underarm hair begins to grow. Like hair at the base of the penis, this hair is usually fine, soft, and lightly colored at first before turning darker and coarser.

Acne

About the same time underarm hair begins to grow, your teen's sweat- and oil-producing glands also start developing. If these glands get clogged up, it can cause acne. I'll talk more about treating acne in chapter 7.

Where the Girls Are

First a word of warning: Puberty is *really* different from girl to girl, and the evidence is revealed in any seventh-grade classroom. Some girls are flat chested, while others show off hourglass figures and décolletage that a Hollywood starlet would pay good money for.

Puberty begins at different times and lasts for different periods of time for each girl. The sequence of puberty from breast development to complete physical maturity may be as short as a year and a half, or the process may take as long as five or—rarely—six years. This open-ended period can be as difficult for girls as it is for boys, especially if their peers have entered or even completed puberty before they've even started.

Nevertheless, it's true that girls typically mature sooner than guys do, entering puberty a year to two years earlier than boys do. It's important to keep this in mind because you need to reassure your children that the only sure thing about puberty is that no two young people go through it alike. I like to compare puberty to an old Model T engine—one that pops and spurts until it begins humming.

Growing Up and Up

Puberty in girls, just as in boys, causes growth spurts, but girls average only about three inches of growth per year. Like boys, your daughter's head, hands, and feet are the first things to grow. Then she'll grow in her arms and legs, and finally her torso, hips, and shoulders will catch up with the rest of her body.

For most girls, growth spurts begin about the age of ten and end when they're twelve. After that, most girls continue to grow, just at a slower pace, until they are seventeen or eighteen.

Five Stages of Puberty for Girls

Here's a timeline used by doctors and developmental experts to help them better understand puberty. It's called the Tanner Classification of development:

Stage 1: From birth until eight to eleven years old—
the average end of this stage is nine to ten years old

In Stage 1, there are no outward signs of sexual development, but your daughter's ovaries are enlarging and hormone production is beginning.

Stage 2: Usually eight to fourteen years old—
the average end of this stage is ten to eleven years old

The first sign of puberty is typically the beginning of breast growth, including breast buds, which doctors call *thelarche*. A girl also begins to grow considerably. The first signs of pubic hair start out fine and straight rather than curly.

Stage 3: Usually nine to fifteen years old—
the average end of this stage is eleven to twelve years old

Breast growth continues and pubic hair coarsens and becomes darker, but there still isn't much of it. Your girl's body is still growing, and her vagina is enlarging and may begin to produce a clear or whitish discharge, which is a normal self-cleansing process. Some girls get their first menstrual periods late in this stage.

Stage 4: Usually ten to sixteen years old—
the average end of this stage is twelve to fourteen years old

Pubic hair growth takes on the triangular shape of adulthood, but it doesn't quite cover the entire pubic area. Underarm hair is likely to appear about two years after pubic hair starts growing. The first period, or what doctors call *menarche*, occurs. Ovulation (the release of egg cells) begins in some girls, but a regular monthly routine doesn't begin until Stage 5.

Stage 5: Usually twelve to nineteen years old—
the average end of this stage is fourteen to fifteen years old

This is the final stage of development when a young girl physically becomes an adult. Breast and pubic hair growth are complete, and full height is usually attained by this point. Menstrual periods are well established, and ovulation occurs monthly. Acne can appear about the same time as underarm hair—just like the boys.

Breasts

Almost invariably, it would shock the fathers of my girl patients to learn that breast development can start as early as seven years of age. Then again, it can begin as late as thirteen years of age, but that's rare these days. Either way, the breasts continue to develop through the end of puberty.

Breast development starts with the enlargement of the flat area around the nipple (areola, or *uh-ree-oh-la*). Some breast tissue forms under the nipple. Breast budding, which may begin on one side before the other, is often accompanied by tenderness that generally goes away after a few months. When breast development is complete—and most of my patients are surprised to learn this—the breasts are usually different sizes. In addition, breast size varies from girl to girl, and there is no natural or safe way for your teen girl to make her breasts larger or smaller other than cosmetic surgery. Breast augmentation is a procedure I don't consider healthy for teens.

The nipple is the exit point of many small ducts that come from the breast glands that produce milk. With rubbing or stimulation, drops of a milky or clear discharge can appear. This is normal. If the discharge comes from only one breast or is bloody, discolored, or pus-like, a doctor should check it out.

FYI . . . ⏪ ▶ ⏸ ⏹ ⏩

▶ Most girls (and their moms) are pleased to learn that breast cancer is incredibly rare during the teen years. Breast lumps, however, are extremely common during adolescence. Teen girls often get cysts or benign growths (tumors) in their breasts, which are caused by hormonal changes. Most of the time, these small lumps disappear on their own, but if they persist over two or three cycles, it's a good idea to have your daughter's doctor take a look.

Pubic Hair

Pubic hair starts along the larger vaginal lips (the labia majora) and becomes darker, coarser, and curlier over time. The development of coarse, dark pubic hair is what doctors call *adrenarche*. Some girls (about 15 percent) will see pubic hair before breast development. The amount of pubic hair increases to an almost adult amount prior to the onset of the menses in some girls. However, most girls don't see an adult amount of pubic hair until closer to the end of puberty.

Acne

Just like boys, when girls begin to grow underarm hair, they begin to develop acne. Your daughter's sweat- and oil-producing glands also start developing. If these glands get clogged up, it can cause acne. I'll talk more about treating acne in chapter 7.

Those Menstrual Periods

The onset of the menstrual cycles (what doctors call *menarche*) begins about two to two and a half years after the onset of breast development. Thus, the menstrual cycle can occur anywhere from age nine to age fifteen and still be considered normal. When periods do begin, they can be very irregular for a year or so. A young girl may skip a month and suddenly experience two periods in twenty-eight days. One month she could bleed heavily; the next month there could be virtually no bleeding. Cramps can come on like gangbusters and not even be noticeable the next time around.

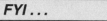

FYI . . .

▶ I've had mothers ask me to prescribe birth control pills (which are essentially strong steroid drugs) to even out their daughter's periods, but rarely is this medically necessary. Furthermore, I have reservations about medicating a normal process, and uneven periods can be a normal process.

For me, the exception would be national-level athletes. For several years, I was a volunteer physician for the U.S. Olympic program, caring for some of our nation's elite athletes. For young women seeking to make the Olympic team or to compete at the highest levels, it made sense to medically manage premenstrual syndrome, cramping, and even regular periods. In those instances, I prescribed low-dose birth control pills that suppressed a woman's period for three to six months. I viewed this as a performance maintainer, not a performance enhancer.

Until the master gland—the pituitary—finds its rhythm, a girl's menstrual cycle may look like a NASDAQ chart with the correlating ups and down. Eventually, the spurts and sputters diminish as the menstrual cycle evens out. This is a message parents should communicate as they take an active role in their daughter's health. And be sure to remind your daughter that periods are part of God's plan—preparing her body to have a baby:

Mandy, your periods are a reminder of God's design. Each month, the womb builds up a lining. If a baby doesn't come that month, the lining sheds and allows a new home to be built the following month. Your body will patiently wait, month by month, until a new baby is conceived.

Puberty is a good time to talk with your daughter about one of the more unpleasant aspects of the menstrual cycle—premenstrual syndrome, also known as PMS. From two to three days to as long as one to two weeks before her period starts, she may feel irritable, become more easily fatigued, and need a little more sleep. When my daughter Kate came of age, she'd sometimes slump over on the couch, fighting yawn after yawn. Barb and I would look at each other, and one of us would say, "Is it that time?" Kate would think for a moment and say, "Yeah, it's been about four weeks."

Check It Out!

▶ There are many good books available to help girls navigate the changes. I recommend *The Period Book* by Karen Gravelle and her niece, Jennifer Gravelle. Another book worth reading is *It's Perfectly Normal* by Robie Harris. These books are written for girls ages nine to thirteen. Find out more about them at my website (www.highly healthy.net).

Asking her in this gentle way helped us anticipate that her cycle was coming, along with the attending cramps. Cramps are no fun, and whenever a young woman would ask me for help finding relief, I usually prescribed a non-steroidal anti-inflammatory drug (NSAIDs). A number of non-prescription NSAIDs are available, including Aleve, Advil, and Motrin I-B. These are all over-the-counter-strength medicines, but you can talk to your daughter's doctor about her taking them in prescription-strength doses. One advantage of Aleve is that it can be taken twice a day; Advil or Motrin has to be ingested three or four times a day. A word of caution: NSAIDs can irritate the stomach, so they are best taken with food.

FYI . . .

▶ *When There Isn't a Growth Spurt*

For some children the engine of growth never turns over. I'm talking about "short stature" children who fall below the 5th percentile on the growth chart. Short stature is often a product of genetics: if teens have short parents, there's a good chance they'll be looking up to their peers for the rest of their lives—and hearing their taunts in school hallways along the way. The Greek philosopher Epictetus declared that "reason is not measured by size of height but by principles," but try selling that to bully-minded kids in the schoolyard.

For children whose short stature is due to a deficiency in growth hormone, a number of companies make a synthetic form of the hormone that can help them grow more normally. One company has suggested limiting the use of synthetic growth hormone to boys who are likely to be shorter than five feet three and to girls likely to be shorter than four feet eleven. Based on current medical knowledge, the use of synthetic growth hormone will allow these children to reach adult heights of up to five feet six in boys and five feet one in girls—much-needed inches that add a dose of self-esteem to short-statured teens. Parents would be well advised to look into growth hormone for the growth hormone–deficient child.

Using growth hormone for genetic short stature, however, is a much more problematic decision that I've counseled many families through. Some studies indicate that people of short stature can face social obstacles. For example, income level and opportunity for career advancement seem to be affected by height. People of both genders who are well below average in height appear to be victims of subtle discrimination. Other researchers believe, however, that these studies are biased and that many children with short stature do not have developmental or social problems.

Nevertheless, many parents believe their child's shortness is a handicap. Because of this widespread belief, some doctors treat short-statured children who have normal levels of growth hormone with the synthetic growth hormone. Injections of growth hormone are not a panacea, and they are extremely expensive. Children must be injected three times a week over a four- to five-year period and might gain only one or two inches of height. This gain in height can cost from $11,000 to $18,000 a year. Before you pursue growth hormone for your preteen or teen who has normal levels of growth hormone, you'd do well to set up an evaluation by a pediatric endocrinologist and a consultation with a psychologist or a pastoral professional.

If you're considering this route, be aware that growth hormone injections are "policy dependent" in terms of medical insurance coverage. Insurance companies require a substantial amount of documentation before approving treatment. (In case you're wondering, they will not, and should not, sign off on growth hormone for children of normal height so they can become the next Shaquille O'Neal or Venus Williams.)

TIMING OF PUBERTY:
ISSUES FOR BOYS AND GIRLS

The differences in the onset and rate of puberty for each boy and girl will definitely affect other areas of their lives. For example, a twelve-year-old girl who has already completed puberty will have interests that are distinctly different from a twelve-year-old girl who hasn't started puberty. That difference is usually spelled b-o-y-s, which means the mature twelve-year-old wants to act like a sixteen-year-old, while the prepubescent twelve-year-old is probably more interested in the things that capture the attention of most ten-year-old girls—like American Doll sets.

Teens who bloom either very early or very late have special concerns. Late bloomers (especially boys) may feel they can't compete in sports with their more physically developed classmates. Early bloomers (especially girls) may be pressured into adult situations—like sexual pressure—before they are emotionally or mentally equipped to handle them. The combined effect of the age when physical changes begin in puberty and the ways in which friends, family, and their world respond to these changes can have long-lasting and potentially life-scarring effects on teens.

On the other side of the coin, some teens like the idea that they're developing differently from their friends—especially if they are early bloomers. There's the attention they garner, and their physical maturity gives them confidence that they're better off than classmates who haven't matured yet. Whatever the rate of growth, however, many teens have an unrealistic view of themselves and need to be reassured that differences in growth rates are normal.

This incredible variation in puberty can cause considerable angst among teens. Just think about it. Suppose your daughter's best friend is six months younger than your daughter, yet this friend is taller, has started having periods, has larger breasts, and has begun to wear a bra. Meanwhile, your daughter is flat as a board and still prefers pigtails. Imagine the horror. Or your son is convinced he's abnormal because his nose looks like a ski ramp and his ears are Dumbo-like, which may be true—for a time—because the features of his face are likely growing up and out at different rates. Egads!

"How I look" was a major worry reported by teens in a 1991–92 University of Wisconsin-Extension Teen Assessment Project. Appearance was the girls' biggest worry (69 percent) and the second biggest worry for boys (45 percent). The study also asked teens how much they worried about whether their bodies were growing normally. Result: they stressed a great deal, although as adolescents got older, they worried less. Half or more of the teens in every grade said they were at least a little worried about this, and girls worried more than boys. Teens' worries were based partly on comparing themselves with their peers. Therefore, early-maturing girls and late-maturing boys risked difficult adjustments because they were the most different from their peers.

Because of all the turmoil surrounding puberty, ignorance is *not* bliss for parents. Long talks before puberty are helpful, but you can play catch-up if you've been virtually silent on this topic. Remember, preteens and teens want the facts, but they'd also love to hear what puberty was like for you. If you can tell stories about how awkward it felt to be shorter than anyone in your class or how embarrassed you were by your acne, by all means share this with your child. Describing your teen experiences—warts and all—will bring you and your son or daughter closer than you've ever been. Be informal. Talk about these things as they arise.

One other point to emphasize: Never compare your teen to a sibling or another child. Comparing your son or daughter to a classmate is unfair and often upsetting for a teen. They develop at such different rates, and that's something they have no control over.

Puberty is one of the most exciting and frightening periods of your teen's life. Your love and support will be more helpful than you could ever imagine. If you take the time and make the effort, you can do a lot to offset the fears and concerns your teen will have about his or her changing body. Here are some tips for easing this process along:

- ❖ Make a conscious effort to look for opportunities to talk about puberty with your preteens and teens. Let them know well ahead of time what changes they can expect.
- ❖ Boys who enter puberty late will need additional support and reassurance—especially from their dads. If the father is not around, then having another significant male speak with your teen boy is critical. Remember, studies show that late-blooming boys worry more than their peers about their development. If you cannot allay your son's concerns, then invite him to talk to a doctor, coach, or youth pastor about physical development.
- ❖ If your son wants to start working out at a gym, consult your teen's doctor about when it's safe to do so.
- ❖ Girls who enter puberty early need additional support and supervision, since early physical maturation can lead to social problems. The

early bloomer may be teased because of precocious physical changes. The older-looking girl is usually expected to act as old as she looks, but her twelve-year-old mind is trapped in a seventeen-year-old body. In addition, her mature appearance often attracts the attention of older boys and increases the likelihood of being befriended by an older peer group—a group more likely to be involved in risk-taking behaviors such as drinking and doing drugs.

❖ Remember that physical development is not related to emotional maturity. Just because a teen looks older doesn't mean he or she is any more mature than the teen who still looks like a little kid. Keep your expectations consistent with your teen's emotional age.

No doubt about it, puberty is a major event in your teen's life—and in yours. Alongside you and your spouse, you'll want another important partner during this remarkable time—your doctor. In the next chapter, we'll look at how to make the transition from a pediatrician to a family physician and why it's important for you, the parent, to remain your teen's health care quarterback.

Chapter 5

FINDING THE RIGHT EXAMINATION ROOM

The faster your child grows, the more often you should beat a path to the doctor's door. Your teen's body, mind, and spirit are undergoing massive changes that need a doctor's trained eye. I've long felt that highly healthy children become highly healthy teens when their parents closely monitor their health and make sure they receive regular checkups throughout the middle school and high school years.

The beginning of puberty is an excellent time to evaluate the issue of your teen's primary care physician. I say this not to tell you to move from one practice to another but to point out that children have different health care needs during adolescence than they do during childhood.

For instance, if your child has been seeing a pediatrician, you may be wondering if it's time to switch to a family physician, internist, or gynecologist. Some pediatricians phase out their adolescent patients by the time they're sixteen, although many are comfortable treating young people up to the ages of eighteen or twenty.

My mother, who was a nurse, knew a good doctor when she saw one, and she believed that Dr. Gloria Weir, a pediatrician, was the best physician for children in our town. Dr. Weir certainly had a way with kids. I never felt embarrassed around her, and I always felt encouraged and affirmed. I'll never forget my last physical with her when I was twenty-one and about to marry Barb. Dr. Weir, bless her heart, put her hands on her hips and said, "Walt, this is the *last* exam I will do for you. We have to cut the cord."

If your teen sees a pediatrician rather than a family physician, you'll have to cut the cord with your pediatrician at some time as well. Adolescent boys often feel awkward around pediatricians, especially female ones, since a routine physical includes a hands-on examination of the penis and testicles. Adolescent girls generally feel awkward and embarrassed putting their legs into stirrups for a pelvic examination by a male doctor.

In addition, many teens feel out of place in pediatric offices, which are often decorated for smaller children. The plastic toys, building blocks, and Dr. Seuss books are dead giveaways. The best time to consider transitioning your child out of a pediatric practice will depend on the pediatrician's comfort with adolescent patients—as well as your and your teen's comfort with the pediatric practice.

Whenever the cord is cut, though, the question becomes, Who should become your teen's new doctor? Many families gravitate toward a respected family physician, and that's how insurance companies like to do things anyway. In the last twenty-five years, as insurance companies attempt to control costs, many have appointed the primary care physician as the gatekeeper into the medical care system. The primary care physician coordinates and oversees your family's health care, referring you to specialists as needed.

LISTEN UP!

Some girls and their mothers prefer to see an obstetrician/gynecologist because they specialize in female care. I understand that reasoning, although I think most young women would do fine with a family physician. While many ob/gyns enjoy providing primary care, there are those who do not. It's also important to discuss with your teen daughter whether she wishes to see a male or female doctor. You as their health care quarterback need to carry out this important task so that your teen remains highly healthy.

Dr. Walt Larimore

IT'S IN THE PLAYBOOK:
QUARTERBACKS AND COACHES

A football analogy is apropos here: you, the parent, need to quarterback your teen's health care. Your health care coach should be a good primary care physician—a medical expert willing to listen to, advise, and sometimes even cajole you. Then there are what I call "game day specialists," or "assistant coaches"—doctors trained in a specific aspect of the health care game. Specialists know almost everything there is to know about a particular part of the body, but they seldom see the entire game the way you and your coach can.

As life marches down the field, you should be—no, make that *will be*—calling the health care plays for your teen. You are still the parent, and while your teen is growing more mature by the month, he or she is far too immature to make many health care decisions—even if the law says she can (I'm speaking about a teen's ability to receive birth control pills or an abortion, for instance, without your consent or even your knowledge). This isn't the time to say it's the doctor's job. You, as a parent, *must* remain your teen's health care quarterback. Sure, at some point—usually late in the teen years or when they leave home and enter college—your role will transition to becoming a mentor, but for now, you need to stay in the game.

Many family physicians won't mind your calling the signals. Even though we've gone to medical school for years and know more about medicine than any layperson can ever hope to know, we understand that *you* know your teen much better than we'll ever know that person. Besides, you love your child with all your heart, and we know that you have his or her best interests at heart. That's why you've brought him or her to our office to receive the best possible medical care.

Your family physician wants to partner with you regarding your teen's health care needs. A good doctor understands that it's his or her job to diagnose your teen's problem, make medical judgments, and then render an opinion in clear English that will help *you* make the final call.

In these days of managed care, acting as your teen's health care quarterback is especially important. You may have noticed that family physicians do not dilly-dally around the examination room. Many spend less time with patients because they have to see so many patients each day to cover their overhead. You may have noticed that insurance companies are dictating what tests and treatments they'll pay for. That's why you need to be intimately involved in the health care of your teens. Our health care system works best when your doctor patiently describes the best options for your teen's health care and then steps back and allows you to make the final decision.

This advice doesn't apply to emergency medical care, when certain conditions require snappy attention from experienced, well-trained ER doctors. When an accident has occurred (which is how most teens end up in an emergency room), you don't have the luxury of discussing a laundry list of medical treatment options. You'll have to focus and listen intently, since decisions must be made on the fly. I hope you'll never have to face any huge medical decisions in an emergency waiting room.

LISTEN UP!

Every good quarterback needs a coach, and this coach is your teen's personal physician. I highly recommend you choose a primary care physician (PCP), such as a family physician or pediatrician who routinely cares for adolescents. Your teen's PCP should work closely with you regarding the medical decisions that must be made. Your coach must take the time to provide—or teach—the critical information you need to know. It's hard to get a doctor to stay in a room long enough, but you must stand your ground and politely ask for this type of care.

Dr. Walt Larimore

The Doctor's Worldview

The doctor's worldview is an important factor to consider. Where does he or she stand on the moral issues of the day—premarital sex, out-of-wedlock pregnancy, drug use, and abortion on demand? Are these views in sync with yours?

Most current consent laws are written to empower the underage teen, not the parents. In one of those "Alice in Wonderland" moments of absurdity, our nation's lawmakers decided that teens under the age of eighteen have the right to ask for and receive birth control prescriptions, be treated for pregnancy, receive treatment for sexually transmitted infections and diseases, and have an abortion without parental notification. Pro-abortion organizations argued that minor teens have a "right of privacy" and a need to make these decisions away from parental "interference." How this happened in a society that won't allow a school nurse to give a ninth-grader two acetaminophen tablets without parental consent is beyond me.

That's why the first thing I, as a parent, would want to know is where my doctor stands on these consent issues. If you believe—as I do—that God holds *parents* responsible for their children's health and well-being, you'll want to partner with a doctor who agrees. Even though your teens may have the legal right to receive—and a doctor may legally provide—certain types of medical care without parental consent, you and the doctor can agree that you will be kept in the loop regarding your teen's health care issues, and both of you can inform your teen of this decision.

On a number of occasions, I've sat in the examination room with a parent and a teen and looked the mother in the eye and said, "Your unmarried daughter can obtain birth control information, birth control pills, treatment for sexually transmitted infections, pregnancy tests, and even an abortion in our state without your knowledge and permission. I want you to know—and I'm telling you this in front of your teen—because I want your daughter to understand that I will not participate in that type of care. If you or she don't agree, you'll have to find another doctor. Is that okay?" The vast majority of parents and teens were very grateful for my blunt language. I took that moment to reiterate that my responsibility, in front of God, was to be a doctor who supported the role of the parent.

Although this type of doctor may be hard to find in your area, it's worth seeking one who shares your point of view. It will take some asking around, but finding the right doctor usually involves some legwork anyway. Word of mouth and personal recommendations are good places to start. Ask your pastor, your friends, and people in your community whose opinions you respect. Are there doctors or nurses in your congregation who can make recommendations? Is there a name or two that keeps cropping up?

Here are some questions you can ask these folks:

- ❖ Have you found a doctor you're comfortable with?
- ❖ What makes him or her a good doctor?
- ❖ Is he or she a good listener?
- ❖ How does he or she feel about prescribing birth control to unmarried teens?
- ❖ Where does he or she stand on abortion?

Selecting the best doctor requires gathering information. Although many insurance companies limit your choices, you can still find a good fit. Think through the following questions because they can make all the difference in the world:

- ❖ Do I want a doctor who is disease oriented or wellness oriented?
- ❖ Do I prefer a conservative or an aggressive approach to care?
- ❖ Would I rather have a doctor who is informal and warm, or formal and detached?
- ❖ Do I prefer a doctor who invites my participation or one who tells me what to do?
- ❖ Do I desire a male or a female doctor?
- ❖ Do I prefer a doctor who is interested in or even supportive of my spiritual interests?

The Doctor's Credentials

Credentials and qualifications are also important benchmarks. Perhaps the top qualification to look for is "board certified." All the primary care specialties for adolescent medicine grant board certification for a specified time, usually seven to ten years. After that, the board certification expires and a physician must undergo another rigorous test. You can certainly ask whether your teen's physician is currently board certified. If he or she is not, you should find the explanation reasonable. For example, some pediatricians and family physicians are bothered by the immense costs associated with taking this exam. Others find it difficult to travel to a distant city to sit for a one- or two-day recertification exam. Physicians who don't want to remain board certified can vouch that they're still involved in quality continuing medical education by obtaining the American Medical Association's Physician's Recognition Award.

In addition, for some specialties (such as pediatrics and obstetrics/gynecology), physicians cannot qualify for board certification until they have been in practice for a specified time. These doctors can say they are board eligible until they pass their board exam.

Background Checks

To further narrow your search, check out the public information about prospective providers that is available through professional organizations like the

Better Business Bureau and your state's department of professional regulation and insurance. Some states have Internet databases that allow you to investigate malpractice cases and complaints, or you can check with the county clerk. You should be able to find out whether a doctor is currently licensed and if the state has ever taken disciplinary action against him or her. Most states allow you to request a copy of the disciplinary order if there have been actions.

Check It Out!

▶ *Examining Your Doctor* by Timothy McCall, M.D., is an excellent resource that shows you how to ask the tough questions to prospective doctors. Learn more about ordering this book at my website (www.highlyhealthy.net).

Keep in mind, however, that anyone who hires an attorney can file a lawsuit at any time. Just because someone filed a lawsuit doesn't necessarily mean a physician is a bad doctor. What you want to look for is a *pattern*. Has this physician been hit with several legal actions in the last few years? If so, it should probably raise a red flag.

The American Medical Association provides information on virtually every licensed physician in the United States on its "Physician Select" website, which you can access through my website (www.highlyhealthy.net). The AMA says that all physician credentials data has been verified for accuracy and authenticated by accrediting agencies, medical schools, residency training programs, licensing boards, and other data sources.

THE FIRST VISIT WITH A NEW DOCTOR

When you visit a doctor's office for the first time, take a look around:

❖ Is it clean and tidy, or does it smell like they failed to use disinfectant the last time someone threw up in the waiting room?
❖ What kind of reading material is in the waiting area? (You can often get a glimpse at the interests of the doctors in the practice by what is sitting out for patients to read.)
❖ Is there a patient educational library with literature available for checking out?

❖ How long did you have to wait to see the doctor? (Some backups are unavoidable, but I always tried to see my patients within fifteen minutes of their scheduled appointment. If I could not, I made sure my staff informed my patients and gave them three choices: (1) wait to see me (the staff would estimate how long it would be), (2) see one of my partners, or (3) reschedule.

When you and your teen get in to see your doctor, have your questions written down. Most doctors don't have time for a lot of chitchat, so they'll welcome hearing your questions or concerns right away—and you'll be demonstrating that you're interested in a doctor-patient relationship that is a win-win. More and more doctors who care for teens are open to hearing these specific questions related to the expectations you have for the management of your child's health care.

Listen to how the doctor responds to you. Does he or she talk down to you? Do you feel like you're being lectured to, or is there a warm bedside manner? How comfortable do you feel in the doctor's presence? Does he or she explain things in layperson's language, or does he or she spout medical jargon?

Taking a doctor's spiritual temperature is easier than you think. Increasingly, doctors are using spiritual inventories (or histories) with their patients. When a doctor inquires about a patient's spiritual beliefs, it opens the door for a parent to ask about a doctor's beliefs and practices related to medical care. If the doctor doesn't employ a spiritual inventory, raise the topic yourself. In a nonthreatening way you might say, "Are you willing to consider my religious and spiritual preferences as you care for my teen?" The doctor will probably ask you what those religious and spiritual preferences are, and you can then ask whether he or she would be willing to work with your spiritual mentors (pastors, priests, rabbis, elders) in the event that your teen is stricken with a serious disease or is involved in a major car accident. If you sense an openness, you may want to inquire if religious faith is a source of strength and comfort to him or her. (Remember, though, that if the doctor is in a group practice, the other doctors in the practice may well answer these questions differently.)

After the office visit, debrief with your teen by asking for his or her thoughts. It's another way to involve them in their own health care. I can remember sitting at the dinner table and talking with Kate when she was around ten or eleven. "Your body is beginning to change," I said to her, "and you're growing older. Ever since you were a little baby, we've taken you to Dr. John [my partner and also a family doctor]. If at any point you feel uncomfortable seeing him, or think you'd rather have a woman doctor than a man doctor, that's A-OK with me. Dr. John will completely understand. Mom and I just want to help you find the best care. Part of growing up is making decisions like this."

Kate appreciated my bringing up the topic, and we had a tender discussion that night. She decided she wanted to continue seeing *her* family physician, Dr. John, and she loved being a patient at our office because she had a great relationship with our nurses and staff. We supported that decision, because we knew it was a good one.

LISTEN UP!

There's no 100 percent right—or wrong—way to go about choosing your teen's doctor. That's why I'd urge you to pray about this decision over several days. It's certainly important enough, right? Asking the Lord of the universe to guide your steps and lead you to the right doctor seems like a very wise thing to do.

Dr. Walt Larimore

TAKING RESPONSIBILITY

Once you've settled in with a family physician, you can switch your focus to long-term health goals. One of the main reasons I wrote this book was to help parents transfer the responsibility of looking after their children's health care onto the shoulders of their teens. By the time they leave home, your teens will thus have a strong foundation for their health care, which, of course has lifelong implications. When you feel crummy, life feels crummy. As any sick person will tell you, "It doesn't feel good to not feel good."

Nonetheless, your teen's health is too important to say, "Missy, you're in high school now, and it's about time you take the responsibility of looking after your body. From this day forth, you're in control of which doctor you see, when you visit a doctor, and what type of care you will receive." I firmly believe parents are not acting wisely if they take this approach.

Instead, a delicate balance must be sought. During the transitional years, parents should begin teaching their teen how to become his or her own health care quarterback—making health care decisions and understanding the consequences of those decisions. I've come across fathers and mothers, though, who've chosen a more laissez-faire approach—looking to their doctor to call the shots—which has ominous repercussions because today's laws allow children to make their own reproductive health care decisions. Parents, therefore, need to maintain a hand on the rudder.

When a teen enters puberty, I recommend that parents schedule an annual physical so that the family physician will have a medical baseline—or history—to refer to on subsequent visits. The annual checkup is the gold standard of highly healthy care.

FYI...

▶ *What about Teen Immunizations?*

Many parents think immunizations ended when their child presented a completed immunization card to begin kindergarten. Wrong!

The tetanus-diphtheria [Td] components of the diphtheria-tetanus-pertussis (DTaP) vaccine children last receive at four to six years of age should be renewed at least every ten years throughout life—starting when a teen is fourteen to sixteen years old. Other vaccines to ask your doctor about are those for hepatitis A, hepatitis B, measles-mumps-rubella (MMR), influenza, pneumococcus, meningococcus, and chicken pox (varicella). For more information on these vaccines, visit my website (www.highlyhealthy.net).

I recommend being current with a chicken pox shot, which can be a dangerous disease. This vaccine works for 85 percent of people, and even if it doesn't prevent chicken pox, it virtually always prevents severe cases and may reduce the risk of developing shingles later in life. Also, young pregnant women who haven't been immunized against chicken pox can expose their unborn baby to the chicken pox virus, which can be devastating to the baby and costly to treat with medication.

Immunization against the influenza virus, whether by flu shot or nasal spray, is a voluntary vaccine I recommend that teens get each fall. The flu vaccine has virtually no side effects, but it can save teens from a nasty bout with the flu. The risk of teens getting the flu is much lower than it is for older people, but an annual vaccine can keep students from missing a week or more of school. (By the way, since 2003 the flu vaccine has been available in a nasal spray, but it's significantly more expensive than the shot. For some needle-adverse teens, it does save a "poke.")

On occasion parents would ask me about a meningitis vaccine for their children who were preparing to go off to college. Increasingly, colleges and universities are requiring a certificate of meningitis vaccination or a signed waiver—especially for students who live in dormitories. Meningitis is a rare disease, but when a child contracts it, the chances of dying are one in five, which is why I recommend getting the vaccine before teens enter their first year of college.

According to the Centers for Disease Control and Prevention, every teen should have the tetanus-diphtheria, varicella (if your teen has not had chicken pox or received the vaccine as a child), MMR (if not completed as a child), and hepatitis B (if not completed in childhood) vaccines. In some areas of the country, additional vaccines are required. The CDC also recommends that all college freshmen receive the meningococcus vaccine.

In my book *God's Design for the Highly Healthy Child,* I discuss a wide variety of vaccine myths parents hear about or are exposed to on the Internet. One of the best Internet sites to access for information about vaccine myths and truths is the Immunization Action Coalition website (the information there is based on a highly recommended book titled *Vaccines: What Every Parent Should Know*). You can link to this website and learn more about this book and the most common vaccine myths at my website (www.highlyhealthy.net).

THE ANNUAL PHYSICAL

If your child is active in sports, he or she will often be required to undergo a sports physical, while parents whose teen has other interests beyond the ball field must be proactive and make an appointment for him or her. In high school, a coach or athletic director sometimes organizes "gang physicals" just before the start of the sports season. While these mass physicals in the school gym or locker room are often free (or have a nominal fee), participating doctors will not have patient histories on hand, and the actual hands-on physical is often rudimentary at best and inattentive at worst.

It's fine to participate in a school-sponsored physical, but it should be viewed as an ancillary checkup. Your teen's doctor has the necessary records and can, in most cases, do a more thorough job. To me a thorough physical means the doctor evaluates immunization status, checks for health risk factors, does a careful physical exam that includes taking blood pressure and listening to the heart, and orders any needed blood tests.

Specific aspects of an annual physical will vary for a boy and a girl.

For Boys

Turn your head and cough. If you're a male, you know exactly what I'm talking about—the doctor's instructions during the physical examination of the male genitalia. These instructions have been standard operating procedure for male physicals dating back for centuries.

When the doctor places a finger against the top of the scrotum and asks the male to "turn your head and cough," he is looking for a hernia, or rupture in the muscles of the abdomen. When the patient coughs, the hernia (if he has one) will press against the doctor's finger.

But there's a second half to this genital exam, and it's much more important because it involves a check for testicular cancer. The doctor reaches down and gently rolls each testicle between his fingers, checking for lumps or tenderness. The examination *is* mildly uncomfortable but not painful. Adolescent boys make nervous jokes about this hands-on procedure, but it's a vital examination that can save lives.

FYI . . .   ◀◀ ▶ ❙❙ ■ ▶▶

► *Self-Exam of the Testicles*

The Testicular Cancer Resource Center provides these tips for conducting a self-exam for testicular cancer:

❖   Examine each testicle with both hands. Place the index and middle fingers under the testicle with the thumbs on top. Roll the testicle gently between the thumbs and fingers—you shouldn't feel any pain when doing the exam. Don't be alarmed if one testicle seems slightly larger than the other. That's normal.

❖ Find the epididymis, which is the soft, tubelike structure behind the testicle that collects and carries sperm. If you are familiar with this structure, you won't mistake it for a suspicious lump. Cancerous lumps usually are found on the sides of the testicle but can also show up on the front. Lumps on the epididymis are not cancerous.

❖ If you find a lump on your testicle, see a doctor, preferably a urologist, right away. The abnormality may not be cancer; it may just be an infection. But if it is testicular cancer, it will spread unless it is treated. Waiting and hoping will not fix anything. Please note that free-floating lumps in the scrotum that are not attached in any way to a testicle are not testicular cancer. When in doubt, get it checked out—if only for peace of mind!

Testicular cancer leaped into the national news when Lance Armstrong beat the deadly disease to the finish line and later pedaled his way to six consecutive Tour de France victories. Lance was blessed indeed, because his testicular cancer had metastasized and he'd been given a less than 40 percent chance of surviving the disease.

If Lance had been my patient when he was growing up, he would have been taught to perform a self-examination for testicular cancer on the first day of each month—preferably during showering or bathing. "When you're washing the scrotum, you should feel the testicles to see if they are the same size," I said to boys in my examination room. "There should be no lumps or bumps, and if you feel something you haven't felt before—like a knot in the testicle or a lump the size of a BB or a pea—you need to see me immediately."

A concerned mother had called in one afternoon. Someone was filling in that day for our receptionist. "I need to bring Mike in to see Dr. Larimore today," exclaimed the mother in an urgent tone.

The office temp looked at our packed schedule but didn't see any way to squeeze him in. "I'm sorry, but our schedule is already full."

"It's an emergency, and I know Dr. Larimore would want to see him."

"Then you should take him to the emergency room."

"No, Dr. Larimore told me that if my son found a lump in his testicles, he wanted to see him *that* day."

The receptionist balked again, but this mom was insistent. Finally, the receptionist called the matter to my attention and asked me what I wanted to do. To me, it wasn't up for discussion. "Have them come to the office right now!" I said.

Within the hour, Mike and his mom were seated in my examination room. Mike's mother apologized for intruding on my afternoon, but I wouldn't hear of it. "You did exactly what I told you to do," I pointed out. "So let's check things out."

Mike, who was about eleven or twelve years old, felt a twinge of embarrassment as he stood up, dropped his pants and underwear, and allowed me to examine his testicles. One felt normal, but I felt a BB-sized lump on the surface of his left testicle.

"Mike, it's amazing you found this," I said as I motioned for him to put his clothes back on. "Whatever I feel is very small, but it's not normal. We need to do a test to see if it's something we should be concerned about." Then I explained that I didn't have the proper equipment—an ultrasound machine—to take a closer look, but we'd find one right away.

I called Byron Hodges, M.D., a urologist to whom I frequently referred patients, and said, "Byron, here's what I've got. A few minutes ago . . ."

"Send him up right now," replied Dr. Hodges. "I'll see him as soon as he gets here."

Byron called me back an hour later, and I could tell by the concern in his voice that it was serious. "All I know is that the ultrasound shows a hard little mass, so I'll need to take him to the operating room to do a biopsy," he said.

That night Byron had removed the boy's left testicle after a biopsy showed testicular cancer. "He should be okay now, but this kid's self-exam may have saved his life," said my colleague.

Think about it: this all transpired in less than eight hours, and that boy's self-examination on the first day of the month very likely saved his life. To this day, I'm amazed he felt the lump because I had a hard time distinguishing it myself. But Mike did what I had instructed him to do, and his preventative self-exam led to a happy ending.

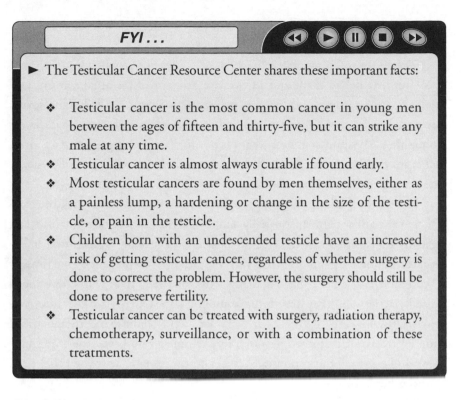

FYI...

▶ The Testicular Cancer Resource Center shares these important facts:

❖ Testicular cancer is the most common cancer in young men between the ages of fifteen and thirty-five, but it can strike any male at any time.

❖ Testicular cancer is almost always curable if found early.

❖ Most testicular cancers are found by men themselves, either as a painless lump, a hardening or change in the size of the testicle, or pain in the testicle.

❖ Children born with an undescended testicle have an increased risk of getting testicular cancer, regardless of whether surgery is done to correct the problem. However, the surgery should still be done to preserve fertility.

❖ Testicular cancer can be treated with surgery, radiation therapy, chemotherapy, surveillance, or with a combination of these treatments.

For Girls

Girls should be seen by their doctors once a year to monitor the physical progress of puberty. Some girls will have an opportunity to get a sports physical at school; for others, parents will need to monitor making the appointments for their physicals.

Girls and Pelvic Examinations

Sooner or later a young woman will have her first pelvic exam and Pap smear. Most young women feel nervous and embarrassed about their first pelvic exam because they've always thought of their genital area as personal and private. It can feel very strange to a girl to have someone examining that part of her body. The purpose of a pelvic exam is to make sure the sexual organs are healthy and working normally. Since most of a female's reproductive organs are inside the body, it's also known as an *internal exam*. These days, it's standard operating procedure to conduct a Pap smear during a routine pelvic exam. The doctor inserts a speculum into the vagina and rubs the cervix with a swab or brush to collect cells that can be checked for cervical cancer. Collecting these cells is painless.

There's an ongoing debate in medical circles about when a girl should have her first pelvic exam and Pap smear. Some medical organizations and many doctors recommend the first pelvic exam after a girl is having sexual intercourse or at twenty-one years of age (some even say eighteen)—whichever comes first. My approach, however, was not to offer a young woman an internal exam or a Pap smear until after she was sexually active—even if it meant she was older than twenty-one.

Here's why I adopted that approach: there is essentially no risk of cervical cancer until a woman is sexually active. Cervical cancer now qualifies as a sexually transmitted disease, and it's caused by a sexually transmitted infection called human papillomavirus (HPV) virtually 100 percent of the time. If a woman who has never been sexually active marries a man who's never been sexually active, and they are mutually monogamous, her risk of cervical cancer is virtually zero. Yet we in the medical field recommend that married women receive Pap smears because there are men who break their marriage vows and don't tell their spouses. A husband can give his wife the HPV virus without her knowing it.

This is how I handled it in my office when a young woman would come in at seventeen or eighteen years of age for her college physical. My nurse, Tish, would say, "There are some doctors who recommend that you have your first Pap smear before you go to college. Dr. Larimore usually recommends that you only have one if you're sexually active. If you're not, we feel it's okay to wait."

At that point the ball was totally in the family's court, and that was fine with me, because the decision to have a pelvic exam should be made by the young woman and her mother. If they wanted to go forward, I respected those wishes. If Mom wanted to stay in the examination room during the procedure, I had no problem with that, but I was happier when moms chose not to stay. One mother told me, "My philosophy about this exam is that it's a rite of passage for my daughter. I have the same reason for not being here for this exam as I would for why I won't be there on her honeymoon." This sounds like a mom teaching her teen to become her own health care quarterback.

Another health care professional should always be in the room with the doctor during a pelvic exam. (I include female doctors in that directive.)

There are a variety of reasons for this:

- ❖ Having a third party in the room increases the likelihood that the visit will remain professional. In those situations where male and female doctors have been accused of molesting a patient, in almost every instance they had performed a pelvic exam alone.

- ❖ The preparation of a Pap smear is done more effectively with an additional set of hands. A second pair of hands is necessary when placing the cervical scrapings on the glass slide, and the glass slide must be set away as quickly as possible to maintain the integrity of the Pap smear.

- ❖ Medical assistants, whether nurses or licensed nurse practitioners, tend to be detail oriented. They are skilled at keeping checklists and following policies and protocol. Having a medical assistant next to me helped me remember to do everything I needed to do during a pelvic exam. On more than one occasion, I heard Tish say, "Don't forget, we were going to do . . ."

- ❖ If a doctor-patient dispute ever reaches the courtroom, and it comes down to a "he said, she said" situation, the patient invariably wins. On the witness stand a doctor testifies, "Of course, I did an internal exam. I did it and wrote down the results." Then the patient testifies that the doctor never touched her. This is often the situation in ovarian cancer and breast cancer malpractice suits. When there's no corroborating witness, the doctor loses every time. And so I teach doctors they should always have breast and pelvic exams witnessed.

I always had my office staff schedule thirty minutes for a young woman's first pelvic exam. It was important to me that it be done slowly, carefully, and sensitively. Before I stepped into the room, I knew Tish had given a fairly extensive explanation of what the exam would entail. She would let the young woman touch the speculum and ask questions. When I came in, I was careful to speak slowly and offer a lot of explanations.

When the time came for the exam, I always turned my back as Tish assisted the young woman onto the examination table. She would scoot her to the bottom of the table and help her place her feet in the stirrup holder, which kept her legs spread apart.

"I have the speculum in my hand," I would say as I showed the young woman the slender tool that looked like a duck's bill. A few minutes earlier,

Tish had placed the speculum under a stream of warm water so it would be warm to the touch. "I'm going to touch your thigh with it," I would say. "Here's what it feels like. Does that feel too warm for you?"

This was a desensitization thing that usually made the young woman feel more comfortable. I would use lubrication with the speculum, but I had to be careful because too much lubrication can mess up a Pap smear. Then I'd gently open the lips of the vagina and slowly slide the lubricated speculum in, looking at the vaginal walls and cervix.

For the Pap smear, I would use a soft brush to rub some cells from the cervix that would be placed in a container of liquid to be sent to a lab for analysis. To test for infections or an STI—since I took nothing for granted in the sexually active woman—I would take a sample of the mucous fluid in the vagina with a soft cotton swab, which would also be sent to the lab. Then I'd place two gloved fingers from my right hand into the vagina and press gently on her abdomen with my left hand to feel the shape and position of her uterus, fallopian tubes, and ovaries. I was looking for lumps or tender spots.

All along, I'd be careful to go very slowly and explain what I was doing and what would happen next. Nothing made me happier than when the young woman said after the exam was finished, "That was easier than I thought it would be!"

Girls and Breast Self-Exams

The female equivalent to a testicular exam is a breast exam, but while testicular cancer tends to strike men in their teens and twenties, the risk of breast cancer increases as women get older. Breast cancer rates spike after women experience menopause; studies show that approximately 80 percent of breast cancers occurs in women age fifty and older.

Breast cancer, then, is rare in young women—very rare. Each year, this deadly disease claims 44,000 lives, but only 200 of those deaths involve women under the age of twenty-five. Nevertheless, I feel it's important for teen girls to develop the habit of examining their breasts on the first day of the month. Some doctors recommend a breast self-examination about five to seven days after menstruation when the breasts are less swollen and tender, but most of my female patients tell me a "first day of the month" pattern is easier to remember.

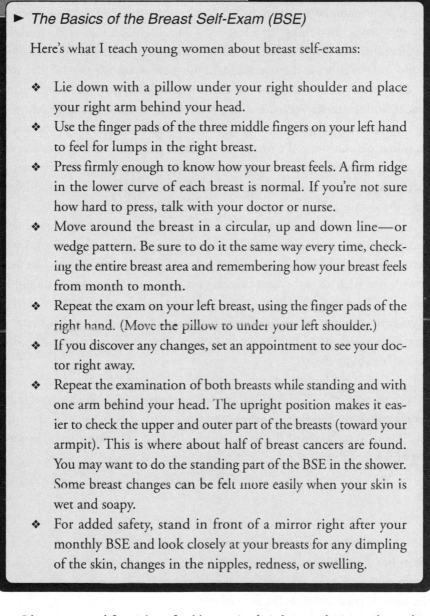

FYI . . .

► *The Basics of the Breast Self-Exam (BSE)*

Here's what I teach young women about breast self-exams:

* Lie down with a pillow under your right shoulder and place your right arm behind your head.
* Use the finger pads of the three middle fingers on your left hand to feel for lumps in the right breast.
* Press firmly enough to know how your breast feels. A firm ridge in the lower curve of each breast is normal. If you're not sure how hard to press, talk with your doctor or nurse.
* Move around the breast in a circular, up and down line—or wedge pattern. Be sure to do it the same way every time, checking the entire breast area and remembering how your breast feels from month to month.
* Repeat the exam on your left breast, using the finger pads of the right hand. (Move the pillow to under your left shoulder.)
* If you discover any changes, set an appointment to see your doctor right away.
* Repeat the examination of both breasts while standing and with one arm behind your head. The upright position makes it easier to check the upper and outer part of the breasts (toward your armpit). This is where about half of breast cancers are found. You may want to do the standing part of the BSE in the shower. Some breast changes can be felt more easily when your skin is wet and soapy.
* For added safety, stand in front of a mirror right after your monthly BSE and look closely at your breasts for any dimpling of the skin, changes in the nipples, redness, or swelling.

It's not unusual for girls to find lumps in their breasts during puberty, but it rarely results in breast cancer at that age. In my years of practice, I can count on one finger the number of teen girls I saw who developed breast cancer—a college coed named Lindsay, who came in complaining about breast pain and a lump she had found during her monthly breast self-exam.

Upon examination, the mass felt harder than the typical lumps I felt in young women. Two things struck me: the lump felt like a small rock, and it was fixed in one place, which meant it didn't freely move. Lumps are often found in fatty tissue and move around a bit. I recommended to Lindsay that we do a biopsy, and I was glad we did. It turned out she had Stage I breast cancer, and the earlier a cancer is detected, the more likely it can be cured.

On another occasion, a family friend named Jamie performed a self-examination and noticed a lump above her left clavicle. She kept an eye on it, checking the mass over the course of the next several days, but it was still there. She showed it to her mom, who said, "I don't know what it is, but let's have the doctor take a look."

I remember the room, I remember what day it was, and I remember what Jamie was wearing—it was one of those days that sticks in your memory. Upon examination, I felt the lump—and it seemed to be a lymph node. "Jamie, I don't know what to say, except this isn't normal. I think the lump should be taken out." A few days later, a surgeon removed the lump, which proved to be a lymphoma, a form of cancer. When cancer is caught that early, the chance of survival is usually high, and I'm happy to report that Jamie has been cancer-free for more than ten years.

College-aged Jamie had been coached well by her doctor and by her parents. It shows how essential your role as a quarterback is during the teen years. It takes work on your part, but no person on earth is better qualified for the job. This is clearly one of the foundational principles for your teens' becoming highly healthy.

One of the most challenging parenting tasks is getting your teen to watch his or her weight. Obesity has become a huge problem in our society, flowing down to the growing ranks of overweight teens. We'll discuss teen obesity in the next chapter, as well as the issue of trying to become *too* fit through the use of anabolic steroids.

Chapter 6

THE CUT LOOK
AND CUTTING LOOKS

With teens' bodies maturing earlier than at any time in human history, I saw some incredibly fit high school athletes in my examination room *and* some incredibly out-of-shape kids who resembled the Pillsbury Dough Boy. Some of the kids dedicated to physical fitness, though, were a little too muscular and had bulked up too much in a very short time for my taste. Their "cut" bodies amazed me. I'm talking about washboard abs, bulging pecs, hulking shoulders, nineteen-inch necks, and buns of steel. And those were the girls! (Just kidding!)

Remember, I had a physical history for many of these kids, with their pubescent past recorded in a chart. If Tish, my nurse, noted that Joe grew from six feet, 180 pounds to six feet one, 210 pounds during the summer break, I seriously contemplated whether Joe was taking anabolic steroids, which are synthetic substances related to the male sex hormones, or androgens. Anabolic steroids promote the growth of muscle size, especially in the chest and shoulders.

THE STEROID SHORTCUT

Gym rats call them "roids," but by any name, anabolic steroids are incredibly effective in bulking up young bodies, adding an extra 15 to 20 percent of lean, hard muscle to the torso. I know—because I once took steroids.

During my freshman year of high school, I was the proverbial ninety-pound weakling, a small fry with a sunken chest. I knew I was a weenie, which was scary to me. I decided to do something about it the summer before my sophomore year. I wanted to bulk up and play football, so I dropped by the gym in Baton

Rouge where many high school football players worked out. As I began pumping my limited amounts of iron, one of the guys running the gym, who could have been Arnold Schwarzenegger's twin, took an interest in me.

"Hey Larimore," he said one day between sets.

"Yes?"

"See these?" he said, holding a small bottle. He poured a couple of dark-colored pills into my right hand. "If you take these, you'll bulk up."

"Really? But aren't they—"

"Don't worry about it. They're completely safe."

So I gulped his little black pills that summer, and that's when I discovered firsthand that his "vitamins" were amazingly effective. My 175-pound rail-thin frame morphed into a Hulk-like 200-pound fighting machine in a single summer. I made the football team, which was terribly exciting, and my new muscular body helped me excel in my main sports—gymnastics and swimming. (By the way, I don't recommend that boys hit the weight room without supervision until puberty has *really* kicked in—usually fourteen years of age in their freshman year of high school.) I continued taking the pills for another year or so, unaware that I was really taking an anabolic steroid called Dianabol. I never had a clue I was doing something dangerous to my body.

How dangerous? Anabolic steroids can affect cholesterol counts, contribute to hardening of the arteries, and take years off your life. Anabolic steroids increase the level of low-density lipoprotein (LDL, or "lethal" cholesterol) and decrease the level of high-density lipoprotein (HDL, or "healthy" cholesterol). High LDL and low HDL levels increase the risk of atherosclerosis, a condition in which fatty substances are deposited inside arteries and disrupt blood flow. If blood is prevented from reaching the heart, the result can be a heart attack; if blood is prevented from reaching the brain, the result can be a stroke. Steroids also increase the risk that blood clots will form in blood vessels, which can also lead to a heart attack or stroke. It's no surprise that studies show that abuse of oral or injectable anabolic steroids is associated with an increased risk for heart attacks and strokes. Most oral anabolic steroids are also associated with an increased risk of severe liver problems, including cancer of the liver. Furthermore, injecting steroids with shared needles or nonsterile injection techniques can cause HIV/AIDS, hepatitis B and C, and bacterial endocarditis.

Most surprising of all, instead of enhancing body image, steroids can do the opposite. In boys and men, the abuse of anabolic steroids can reduce sperm production, shrink the testicles, and cause impotence and irreversible breast enlargement. Girls and women can develop more masculine characteristics, such as deepening of the voice and excessive body hair. In both sexes, anabolic steroids can cause acne and hair loss.

These steroid side effects can occur with any of the anabolic steroids. Steroid abusers, however, often "stack" the drugs—taking two or more kinds of anabolic steroids, mixing oral and injectable types, and sometimes even including compounds designed for veterinary use. Abusers think the different steroids interact to produce a greater effect on muscle size than the effects gained by each drug individually, a theory that hasn't been tested scientifically but dramatically increases the risk of side effects.

Steroid abusers will often "pyramid" their doses in cycles of six to twelve weeks. At the beginning of a cycle, the teen starts with low doses of the drugs being stacked and then slowly increases the doses. In the second half of the cycle, the doses are slowly decreased to zero. This is sometimes followed by a second cycle in which the person continues to train but without drugs. Abusers believe that pyramiding allows the body time to adjust to the high doses, and the drug-free cycle allows the body's hormonal system time to recuperate. As with stacking, however, the benefits of pyramiding and cycling have not been substantiated scientifically.

You won't be able to tell your kids that steroids don't work. They *do* work but at a high cost. Besides potential heart problems and liver cancer, more imme-diate are the psychiatric side effects that cause steroid users to act out aggres-sively and recklessly. Steroids provoke manic symptoms, such as aggression, euphoria, grandiose beliefs, reckless behavior, and a decreased need for sleep. This type of steroid-induced behavior has been given a name—"roid rage."

Frighteningly, the Monitoring the Future study, an annual survey of drug abuse among middle and high school students across the country, showed a significant increase from 1998 to 1999 in anabolic steroid abuse among mid-dle schoolers. During the same year, the percentage of twelfth graders who believed that taking these drugs causes "great risk" to health declined from 68 percent to 62 percent.

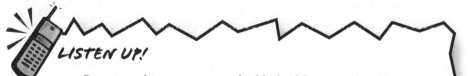

LISTEN UP!

Parents seeking to nurture highly healthy teens should address steroid use head-on, especially if they have athletic children. Point out the dangers. Print off research results from websites such as the National Institute on Drug Abuse. Remind them that steroids can cut decades from their life span.

Dr. Walt Larimore

THE TRUTH ABOUT SUPPLEMENTS

The same song can be sung for dietary supplements like creatine, the now-banned ephedra, and androstenedione (more commonly known as "andro"). There's virtually no data that any of these supplements do any good, although some evidence says creatine may give sprinters a sudden burst of energy. Each of these supplements, however, has significant side effects—including death. The baseball world was shocked in early 2003 when Baltimore Orioles pitcher Steve Bechler—an ephedra user—died of a heatstroke during a spring training workout. Bechler's body temperature had risen to 108 degrees, causing his major organs to fail. Toxicology tests on Bechler revealed significant amounts of ephedra in his blood, and the dietary supplement was a factor in causing the heatstroke that led to his death, according to the Broward County (Florida) medical examiner. In a related premature death, attorneys for the Minnesota Vikings claim that ephedra contributed to Kory Stringer's death from heatstroke in 2001.

Sadly, there hasn't been a quick condemnation of these substances by many sports organizations. When slugger Mark McGwire freely admitted he used androstenedione while setting baseball's single-season home run record in 1998, he wasn't kicked out of the game or stripped of his achievement. I'm now pleased to note that Major League Baseball, the International Olympic Committee, the National Football League, the National Basketball Association, the National Collegiate Athletic Association, the Association of Tennis Professionals, and most high school athletic associations have banned the use of androstenedione.

Parents are on their own when it comes to separating the wheat of dietary supplements from the chaff of bogus manufacturers' claims. Because of a 1994 federal law known as the Dietary Supplement Health and Education Act (DSHEA), the federal government, which leaves the American consumer exposed to the moral turpitude of the manufacturer, does not regulate dietary supplements. This explains why herbs, vitamins, and supplements purchased off the shelf, through direct mail, and on shopping channels are often advertised with wild claims aimed at an unsuspecting public:

❖ incredible fat-loss pill
❖ double your strength in just one month
❖ blow the doors off against your opponents

Not only are these claims unproven, 25 percent of the time the dietary supplements don't have the ingredients they're purported to contain. Consumer

Lab.com, an independent quality-testing laboratory, has tested more than eight hundred supplements and found that between 30 and 40 percent of herbs contain substances—in some cases, toxic—that shouldn't be there. Twenty percent of vitamins aren't the real deal either. In other words, you may think you're buying 500mg pills of Vitamin C with rose hip, but 20 percent of those pills contain other potentially dangerous substances. Without independent quality testing, you have no way of knowing this.

Here's the bottom line on growing bodies: children whose weight and height are in the normal range can't safely do much on their own to accelerate their growth and development. God designed them the way they are. Supplements and vitamins do almost nothing to speed this process along; indeed, they can be harmful. A balanced diet, exercise, and weight lifting helps a young person build muscle, but that's always been the case.

Check It Out!

▶ I urge you to check out ConsumerLab.com, which is a great source for unbiased testing information to help in the selection of better quality nutritional products. You can print off a list of specific products that have passed quality testing and then buy the least expensive product on the list. One-year access to the ConsumerLab.com website has a subscription cost—well worth the peace of mind, but most of the information is available at no cost on my website (www.highlyhealthy.net).

The Natural Medicines Comprehensive Database (check it out at www.naturaldatabase.com) reviews over 4,500 herbs, vitamins, and supplements. You can use their search engines to view the label of any dietary supplement sold in the U.S. and learn more about the listed ingredients. This subscription site is much more expensive than Consumer Lab.com, but the patient version is available at no cost via my website (www.highlyhealthy.net).

Finally, I've coauthored a book titled *Alternative Medicine* that can help parents and teens make wise, evidence-based decisions about alternative therapies, herbs, vitamins, and supplements.

MAJOR LEAGUE EXPANSION

At the other end of the physical-fitness spectrum, more teens than ever are soft around the middle—"couch potatoes" who park themselves in front of the TV with one hand gripping the channel flipper and the other dipping into a bowl of potato chips. The prevalence of obesity among children has reached epidemic proportions in this country with approximately 15 percent of U.S. adolescents considered obese, meaning they weigh at least thirty to forty pounds above their ideal body weight. In all, around one-quarter of America's youth are overweight, and in some states it's 30 to 40 percent of kids.

Jimmy was a typical example—a fourteen-year-old who was five feet six inches tall. When I entered the examination room, Tish handed me his chart. What leaped off the page was his weigh-in—194 pounds.

After exchanging pleasantries, I commented, "Jimmy, you're overweight, right?"

"Yeah, Doctor," he said sheepishly. "I guess I have a few extra pounds."

"Do you know how overweight you are?"

"Twenty pounds?"

"Have a look at the chart," I said, pointing to his growth chart. "Here's how you've grown over the last four years. And now you're twenty-four pounds above the upper limits for normal for your age. How old are you again, Jimmy?"

"Fourteen."

"You've still got some growing to do. If you don't gain another pound between now and eighteen, you'd be normal weight at eighteen. What I'm saying is that you don't have to drop much weight now, but if you're interested in having a normal weight, you need to make some changes now so you can reach your goal. Do you want me to help you?"

"Yeah."

"It'll take more than just you and me working on this. It will also take your family. Let's schedule a time when you and your mom and pop and your brother can come in. I'll spend some time with you first, and then we'll have a dietician meet with your family. It'll probably take about an hour. We'll want to find out what you guys are eating, what your lifestyle is like, what things you like to do, and what things you don't like to do. We'll design a program for your whole family."

My view is that overweight kids are more a manifestation of a family problem than an individual problem. In other words, couch potatoes are not born; they are grown. This view is buttressed by an ACNielsen survey in which parents correctly blamed themselves—not genetics—for their children's obesity, with fast-food restaurants coming in a distant second.

This is really quite encouraging, because when parents take charge of their children's fitness, kids' pounds start shedding like wool sweaters on a warm spring afternoon. Parents are the key to helping control what their children eat and how much they exercise. Jean Wiecha, a senior research scientist at the Harvard School of Public Health, says this kind of involvement is crucial: "[Parents] can create an environment at the home that encourages good health by having an assortment of healthy foods around, by making sure that there are limits set on television, and by having meals as a family in the evening."

This can mean simple things like serving more nutritious meals and smaller portions, serving water or fat-free milk instead of soft drinks at family mealtimes, and limiting or eliminating bad fats and bad sugars. Changing long-standing family eating habits involves some parental discipline, however. Busy parents are often loath to restrict what their children eat because they feel guilty for working so much. Taking the family out to Pizza Hut during the week and letting the kids order an extra-large Stuffed Crust Gold pizza is viewed as a treat. But when hungry teen boys chow down on three slices, they've just ingested 1,580 calories and eighty-one grams of fat. And an ice cream sundae at Baskin-Robbins is often sure to follow.

This mind-set can and should change. I remember seeing a family whose father and mother were extremely overweight. Their son Robbie was obese and had asthma and knee pain. The other two children were in poor shape and wrestling with depressive disorders.

"This is all changeable," I announced that afternoon to the mother. "It's not Robbie who has to change but the whole family."

The mother nodded, and I noted a look of determination on her face. She met in my office with a dietician, who showed her how to fill out a food diary. We've discovered over time that the average family eats the same nine or ten meals for dinner each month—fried chicken, hamburgers, sausage, hot dogs, and pizza. The dietician looked at their diary and suggested replacing a fried chicken meal with something healthier—like baked chicken sprinkled with herbs and spices. Take-out pizza could be replaced by a healthy homemade version.

And so it went. The food diary kept the family accountable, and over the next six months, they made wholesale changes to their nutrition—more home-cooked meals, less McDonald's on the run. They cut way back on their sweets. They began walking as a family before supper, which increased metabolism and in a strange way made them less hungry. The entire family slimmed down within two years. Robbie's knees stopped bothering him, and his breathing improved. When his sister's depressive disorder stabilized, this family became one of the real success stories in my practice.

LISTEN UP!

I hate to be the bearer of bad news, but a lifetime of cheeseburgers, crispy chicken sandwiches, thick-crust pizza, carnitas burritos, garlic fries, and thick chocolate shakes will make you as fat as the Goodyear blimp.

Nick Yphantides, M.D., *author of*
My Big Fat Greek Diet, *who once weighed 467 pounds*

Obesity Takes a Toll Emotionally

Obesity during the teen years can yield emotional and social trauma as well, especially from the court of public opinion—their peers. Chubby teens are often teased and bullied by their classmates, which can lead to low self-esteem. Obese children can feel as low as teen cancer patients do. In 2003, University of California researchers compared quality-of-life scores of obese children with those of normal-weight, healthy children and with children who were undergoing chemotherapy. Obese children were nearly six times more likely to report an impaired quality of life than healthy, normal-weight children. Even more shocking, severely obese children rated their quality of life as about the same as children with cancer who had been treated with chemotherapy!

A University of Minnesota study found a strong association between the teasing endured by overweight teens and rates of depression, low body satisfaction, low self-esteem, and eating disorders. "Of particular concern," wrote study author Marla Eisenberg, "are the alarming rates of suicidal ideation [thinking of committing suicide] and attempts associated with weight-based teasing, which are two to three times as high among those who were teased compared with those not teased."

Raising highly healthy teens requires making the effort to serve highly healthy meals. Not only will your teens' waistlines notice the difference, but their self-esteem will as well.

Check Out Those BMIs

The height-weight charts I've used in practice for more than twenty years are headed for the trash bin. The American Academy of Pediatrics recommends that physicians no longer flip to the height-weight charts for children between the ages of two and twenty but instead use the Body Mass Index (BMI) as the standard assessment tool. Physicians and researchers who study obesity find the BMI to be their measurement of choice. Thus, parents should get clued in quickly about BMIs.

The BMI uses a mathematical formula that takes into account a person's gender, height, and weight. As a strict formula, the Body Mass Index equals a person's weight in kilograms divided by height in meters squared. For you slide-rule types, that's BMI = kg/m^2. I can hear you saying, "This is America, and we use feet and inches to measure height and pounds to measure weight." You can find a converted Body Mass Index chart on page 126.

Any number between 19 and 24 is considered normal, but BMIs of 27 or 28 are where researchers say they begin to see a greater risk of diabetes, cardiovascular problems, hypertension, osteoarthritis, and certain cancers. The Centers for Disease Control notes that children born today carry a 33 percent chance of developing diabetes—even higher in the African-American and Hispanic populations.

It's never too late for a course correction. Whenever chubby children with BMIs in the thirties came into my practice, I would view them as I'd view smokers. In other words, I wanted them and their parents to be aware of the long-term health risks associated with being overweight and obese. How successful were my interventions? I probably turned around 20 percent of families—not a high number. What decisions will you make today about your family's weight?

LISTEN UP!

Obese teens have significantly more difficulty losing and maintaining weight loss because their physical condition has dramatically increased the number and the size of their fat cells. Obese teens may have up to five times more fat cells than lean teens. Here are the ramifications: You don't lose these fat cells when you lose weight. Weight loss will cause a decrease in fat cell size but not in fat cell number. Part of raising highly healthy teens, then, is preventing them from becoming overweight or obese in the first place.

Dr. Walt Larimore

BODY MASS INDEX TABLE

BMI	Normal						Overweight					Obese										Extreme Obesity														
	19	20	21	22	23	24	25	26	27	28	29	30	31	32	33	34	35	36	37	38	39	40	41	42	43	44	45	46	47	48	49	50	51	52	53	54
Height (inches)												Body Weight (pounds)																								
58	91	96	100	105	110	115	119	124	129	134	138	143	148	153	158	162	167	172	177	181	186	191	196	201	205	210	215	220	224	229	234	239	244	248	253	258
59	94	99	104	109	114	119	124	128	133	138	143	148	153	158	163	168	173	178	183	188	193	198	203	208	212	217	222	227	232	237	242	247	252	257	262	267
60	97	102	107	112	118	123	128	133	138	143	148	153	158	163	168	174	179	184	189	194	199	204	209	215	220	225	230	235	240	245	250	255	261	266	271	276
61	100	106	111	116	122	127	132	137	143	148	153	158	164	169	174	180	185	190	195	201	206	211	217	222	227	232	238	243	248	254	259	264	269	275	280	285
62	104	109	115	120	126	131	136	142	147	153	158	164	169	175	180	186	191	196	202	207	213	218	224	229	235	240	246	251	256	262	267	273	278	284	289	295
63	107	113	118	124	130	135	141	146	152	158	163	169	175	180	186	191	197	203	208	214	220	225	231	237	242	248	254	259	265	270	278	282	287	293	299	304
64	110	116	122	128	134	140	145	151	157	163	169	174	180	186	192	197	204	209	215	221	227	232	238	244	250	256	262	267	273	279	285	291	296	302	308	314
65	114	120	126	132	138	144	150	156	162	168	174	180	186	192	198	204	210	216	222	228	234	240	246	252	258	264	270	276	282	288	294	300	306	312	318	324
66	118	124	130	136	142	148	155	161	167	173	179	186	192	198	204	210	216	223	229	235	241	247	253	260	266	272	278	284	291	297	303	309	315	322	328	334
67	121	127	134	140	146	153	159	166	172	178	185	191	198	204	211	217	223	230	236	242	249	255	261	268	274	280	287	293	299	306	312	319	325	331	338	344
68	125	131	138	144	151	158	164	171	177	184	190	197	203	210	216	223	230	236	243	249	256	262	269	276	282	289	295	302	308	315	322	328	335	341	348	354
69	128	135	142	149	155	162	169	176	182	189	196	203	209	216	223	230	236	243	250	257	263	270	277	284	291	297	304	311	318	324	331	338	345	351	358	365
70	132	139	146	153	160	167	174	181	188	195	202	209	216	222	229	236	243	250	257	264	271	278	285	292	299	306	313	320	327	334	341	348	355	362	369	376
71	136	143	150	157	165	172	179	186	193	200	208	215	222	229	236	243	250	257	265	272	279	286	293	301	308	315	322	329	338	343	351	358	365	372	379	386
72	140	147	154	162	169	177	184	191	199	206	213	221	228	235	242	250	258	265	272	279	287	294	302	309	316	324	331	338	346	353	361	368	375	383	390	397
73	144	151	159	166	174	182	189	197	204	212	219	227	235	242	250	257	265	272	280	288	295	302	310	318	325	333	340	348	355	363	371	378	386	393	401	408
74	148	155	163	171	179	186	194	202	210	218	225	233	241	249	256	264	272	280	287	295	303	311	319	326	334	342	350	358	365	373	381	389	396	404	412	420
75	152	160	168	176	184	192	200	208	216	224	232	240	248	256	264	272	279	287	295	303	311	319	327	335	343	351	359	367	375	383	391	399	407	415	423	431
76	156	164	172	180	189	197	205	213	221	230	238	246	254	263	271	279	287	295	304	312	320	328	336	344	353	361	369	377	385	394	402	410	418	426	435	443

LIVING TO EAT WELL

The principles of good nutrition sound a lot like what Grandma used to say: eat plenty of fruits and veggies, don't snack on junk food between meals, and watch your desserts. Sometimes, however, the spirit is willing but the body isn't, because our country has been incredibly blessed by God with a bounty of food. Compared to what our forefathers had to pay to put meals on the table, it's downright inexpensive too.

Eating is one of life's joys. Instead of eating to live, however, we live to eat. A saturation of fast-food advertising and around-the-clock cooking shows on the Food Network has turned us into a nation that loves food high in fat, low in nutrients, and rich in chocolate. In the battle of the bulge, health is fighting a losing battle. Americans may talk healthy, but we eat tasty.

Good nutrition must start with parents. Kids don't typically cook their own meals, so they eat—or get used to eating—what they're served by you. Preparing nutritious meals takes effort and can tax any household, especially one in which both parents work outside the home. But I can think of no other area of your teen's physical health that can be dramatically influenced every day by a conscientious parent intent on serving healthy meals and snacks to his or her children. Your commitment to the program means you can't fry up a country chicken, prepare mashed potatoes and gravy, and drench lima beans in butter for yourself while serving your teens lean turkey breast and sliced carrot sticks. You have to eat what they eat—and chances are it's best for you too.

When Barb and I reached our forties—while Kate and Scott were young teens—we all realized our readings on the bathroom scales were higher than we cared to admit. One night we sat down to discuss the issue over dinner (no irony intended). We agreed we weren't exercising enough, eating way too much fast food that was high in saturated fats, and failing to resist high-sugar desserts. Just as disconcerting was the fact that our family had been eating more meals while watching television instead of sitting together at the dinner table. We needed to make adjustments, and the first steps were to turn off the TV and start keeping a daily diary of what we were eating.

The results were illuminating. After tracking when, where, and what we ate for one month, we discovered we ate only nine dinners together as a family. Breakfasts were routinely skipped, and soft drinks and chips kept us going between meals. Barb and I agreed things had to change, so we read several how-to books on good nutrition. I don't remember having had a course in basic nutrition—not even in medical school! We beefed up our knowledge about the differences between fats, carbohydrates, and proteins. We learned which snacks were high in dangerous saturated fats, or trans fats.

It's shocking, but fewer than 1 percent of teens in the United States eat what could be considered a healthy diet—the recommended quantities of good foods such as whole grains, vegetables, fruits, and low- or no-fat dairy foods! It wasn't until Barb and I did our own research that we learned to recognize the difference between "good" and "bad" calories.

Diets high in bad carbohydrates include simple or processed sugars (soft drinks, candy bars, and doughnuts) and starches (white rice, white bread, potatoes, most packaged cereals, most pasta, and most baked goods). The body quickly absorbs these foods, which raises the body's blood sugar (glucose) so that the pancreas produces higher-than-normal levels of a hormone called insulin to bring the blood sugar down to normal. At higher levels, insulin increases the accumulation of fat, and excess fat causes insulin resistance, which results in blood sugars being converted to fat and can lead to obesity, type 2 diabetes, heart disease, and blood circulation problems. In addition, bad carbohydrates leave the stomach more quickly than do foods high in fiber, good fats, and proteins, thereby causing hunger to occur earlier than it should.

Let me use a real-world situation to describe how this looks. Teens who eat a sugarcoated cereal soaked in high-fat milk for breakfast become hungry two hours later—right around third hour in school. So they look for something to snack on between classes. Typically their only option is a vending machine, which is available to students in 98 percent of American high schools.

Vending machine foods are Exhibit 1A for every bad carbohydrate, bad fat, and high-calorie carbohydrate food or drink in the book. Soft drinks, candy bars, bags of cookies, and chips are yet again digested and processed quickly by their bodies. Net result: they're ravenous by lunchtime. In the cafeteria, most schools serve more "bad" foods—highly processed fare like pizza, hot dogs, hamburgers, and fries high in saturated fat. More syrupy soft drinks or fruit juices wash down their lunch.

Just as there are bad carbohydrates, there are bad fats. Bad fats cause hardening of the arteries, heart disease, strokes, and many other health problems. The first group is the saturated fats, which are found in milk products (except skim or nonfat milk) and fatty red meat (and to a lesser extent in pork and chicken). A second category of bad fats is the trans fatty acids, which are called "trans fats" by the media. While this book was being written, the Food and Drug Administration was debating whether to require trans fats to be listed on nutrition labels. Until that happens, the presence of these dangerous fats is hidden from the consumer. (Until nutrition labels indicate whether trans fats are present, look for the word *hydrogenated* on the label. Hydrogenated oils are trans fats, and no amount of trans fat is healthy in a diet.) Trans fats are found nearly everywhere, including in margarine, vegetable shortenings, most snack foods, highly processed foods, and baked goods.

FYI...

► U.S. Department of Agriculture data show that the diets of most children are low in many nutrients, especially vitamins E and B6 and the minerals zinc, calcium, and iron. Data from a 1998 survey of more than 5,500 American children showed a rise in snack and soft-drink consumption and a decline in milk consumption. The average child or teen now consumes as much as sixty-five gallons of soft drinks each year. No wonder our teens aren't getting the nutrition they need!

Turning the Ship Around

It's never too late to teach our teens to eat correctly, but turning a family's nutritional ship is like turning a U.S. Navy aircraft carrier around—it's going to take some time. The way Barb and I saw it, though, if we didn't begin implementing the necessary changes, our family's nutritional ship would never get going in the right direction. We had to get our command deck in order before we could tackle the rest of the ship.

At our next family meeting, we told our kids we were going to exercise more—and they were too. We said we were going to eat far fewer dinners in front of the TV. We said we'd be pickier in what we chose to eat. We'd go to bed earlier. I'm happy to report that we did change the direction of our family's nutritional ship, but Barb and I made the mistake of trying to make a quick turn instead of taking a more leisurely tack. I still remember Kate calling Barb's new cooking plan "The Diet of Death." She didn't find it easy to stop eating those good-tasting bad fats and bad sugars.

Barb and I wish we had initiated these changes when our children were younger. Many mothers and fathers feel this way. A national survey of parents indicated that about 70 percent want their children to have good nutrition and eating habits, but only 40 percent said they'd succeeded in this area of parenting. Why the discrepancy between desire and success? Most parents, from what I saw in my practice, weren't willing to practice what they preached (I include Barb and me in that group). If we want our children to be highly healthy, we must model good nutrition and eating habits. If we don't model healthy nutritional habits, our children are destined to a lifetime of being overweight.

PRINCIPLES TO EAT BY

Here are my principles of good nutrition for parents and their teens:

1. Don't Let Your Teens Skip Breakfast

Call us June and Ward Cleaver, but Barb and I made it a point to have a sit-down breakfast with Kate and Scott. For us, cereal and fruit usually sufficed, but sometimes I'd whip up whole-wheat French toast or Barb would make veggie omelets. It didn't matter—it was our family time.

Breakfast is the most important meal of the day. The body's metabolism needs a booster shot when young bodies wake up because they've been dormant all night. When a teen's body doesn't get some food in the morning, it turns to its own muscle mass—not stored fat—for energy. The body's metabolism slows down even more, which explains why teachers can tell during first hour who has eaten and who hasn't. Teens are less likely to skip breakfast when there's good food to eat when they wake up, and they'll tend not to compensate later in the day by overeating.

2. Encourage Your Teens to Eat a Healthy Snack between Meals

To keep the body's metabolism burning and prevent a drop in blood sugar, teens shouldn't let too many hours pass between meals. A low blood-sugar level can leave them feeling sleepy in class and craving sweets. Eating a healthy snack—an apple, banana, or some type of energy bar—can elevate their mood, improve their concentration, and increase their ability to handle stress. Buying a bag of Doritos or Skittles from the vending machine won't cut it.

3. Watch Those Calories and Fat Grams for Your Teens

One of the best government programs of the last twenty years has been the "Nutrition Facts" label on food items sold in the United States. The labels break down a serving size by calories, total fat, cholesterol, sodium, protein, and so forth. These distinctives give parents real direction. The average American consumes 3,000 calories a day but needs less than 2,000. Government dietary guidelines recommend that people get less than 30 percent of their daily calories from fat. Another guideline is that we should eat foods that average three grams of fat for every hundred calories. If a teen eats a double-deck fast-food hamburger with special sauce, he or she will be ingesting a burger that has 40 percent to 50 percent of its calories from fat. The meal should be balanced by something low in fat, like salad with low-fat dressing or a piece of fruit.

It may sound complicated, but losing weight is actually a simple equation: eat fewer calories and exercise more. Works every time it's tried!

4. Educate Your Teens about Better Choices in Fast Food

One-fourth of the U.S. population—70 million people—step inside the doors of a fast-food restaurant every day. This being the case, it shouldn't surprise anyone that probably *half* the teen population is chowing down on chalupas, cheeseburgers, and chili dogs every single day.

It's not realistic to ban your kids from fast-food restaurants, but you can teach them how to order smarter. Fast-food chains, which have been fending off lawsuits from obese people who claim they didn't know fast food would make them fat, are scrambling to offer low-fat, low-carbohydrate, and low-calorie items. What, pray tell, could these food items be? Good question—it's usually some sort of salad or low-fat sandwich.

Teens who drench their salad with regular ranch dressing, however, aren't doing themselves a bit of good; there are around 15 fat grams (20 percent of the daily total) in one serving. Low-calorie or no-calorie dressings are much better for them (although I agree that "no calorie" often means "no taste"). But be aware: some fast-food salads contain more calories and fat grams than burgers. For example, a taco salad at Taco Bell has 380 calories and 42 fat grams because the greens and tomatoes arrive in a fried flour taco shell.

If you're looking for healthier alternatives, pita sandwiches and broiled chicken sandwiches are better choices. Quiznos, Subway, and Schlotzsky's Deli arc national chains that have stepped up with chicken and turkey sandwiches that average 6 grams of fat, and pita sandwiches are making headway as well.

Tell your teens that anything with chicken as the meat ingredient typically contains less fat and fewer calories than the beef versions. Even pizzas dotted with pieces of chicken have roughly half the fat of a pepperoni or Italian sausage version. Stay alert, though: crispy chicken sandwiches and fried chicken pieces contain considerably more fat grams than baked or broiled chicken. The crispy chicken is finger-lickin' good, but as the saying goes, a moment on the lips can mean a lifetime on the hips.

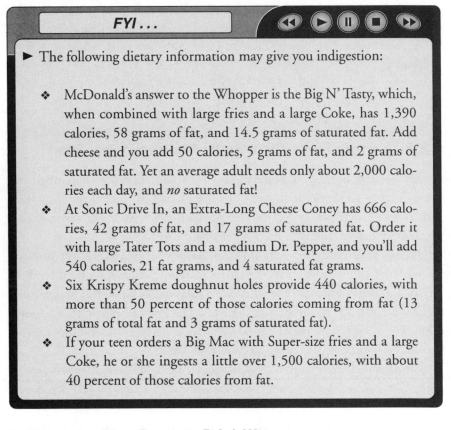

FYI . . .

► The following dietary information may give you indigestion:

❖ McDonald's answer to the Whopper is the Big N' Tasty, which, when combined with large fries and a large Coke, has 1,390 calories, 58 grams of fat, and 14.5 grams of saturated fat. Add cheese and you add 50 calories, 5 grams of fat, and 2 grams of saturated fat. Yet an average adult needs only about 2,000 calories each day, and *no* saturated fat!

❖ At Sonic Drive In, an Extra-Long Cheese Coney has 666 calories, 42 grams of fat, and 17 grams of saturated fat. Order it with large Tater Tots and a medium Dr. Pepper, and you'll add 540 calories, 21 fat grams, and 4 saturated fat grams.

❖ Six Krispy Kreme doughnut holes provide 440 calories, with more than 50 percent of those calories coming from fat (13 grams of total fat and 3 grams of saturated fat).

❖ If your teen orders a Big Mac with Super-size fries and a large Coke, he or she ingests a little over 1,500 calories, with about 40 percent of those calories from fat.

5. Encourage Your Teens to Drink Water, and Then Drink More Water

I have to hand it to soft-drink manufacturers. When teens are thirsty, they're convinced they have to reach for a bottle or can of soda pop. That's the power of television advertising for you.

What about drinking plain old tap water? Teens think that's for nerds. The clear, colorless liquid doesn't have a kick like Mountain Dew, Surge, and Jolt, all of which deliver a caffeine punch—ninety-two milligrams per twenty-ounce drink, or the equivalent of a five-ounce cup of brewed coffee. Yet caffeine causes nervousness, irritability, and restlessness, which means teachers must contend with caffeine-hopping kids immediately following the lunch bell. That's after trying to get them to open their eyes during first hour.

This is a battle in which you, the parent who is seeking to nurture highly healthy teens, must prevail. Water plays an essential role in maintaining health by regulating body temperature, carrying nutrients and oxygen to cells, cushioning joints, protecting organs and tissues, removing toxins, and maintaining strength and endurance. Young people need *more* fluids than adults, for the simple reason that their bodies are still growing. Fluids in the blood transport glucose to the muscles and carry away lactic acid. Fluids in urine eliminate waste products from the body. Fluids in sweat dissipate excess heat and cool the body.

Your teens don't have to drink only water. They can also quaff sports drinks such as Gatorade and Allsports, fruit juices, and nonfat milk. Sports drinks are a mixture of water, a carbohydrate source such as glucose or sugar, and a touch of electrolytes, primarily sodium and potassium. But you really can't improve on fresh, cool water, which God invented for us. Drinking water is habit forming, so help your teens gain a habit to last a lifetime.

6. Wean Your Teens Off Whole Milk

Vitamin D whole milk is rich in taste and rich in fat, but parents have several low-fat versions to choose from: 2 percent, 1 percent, 1/2 percent, and skim milk (no fat). Don't expect your kids to go from whole milk to skim milk in a weekend. We began by putting out 2 percent milk with their breakfast cereal. Barb and I heard a few complaints from the cheap seats, but we didn't back down. A month later, Barb began buying 1 percent milk. It went over okay, but we knew skim milk would be a tougher adjustment, so Barb mixed 1 percent and skim together for a few weeks. After a couple more months, we made the final transition to skim milk. (I must admit, however, that Barb was a bit sneaky about it. She kept the low-fat milk in the full-fat milk container. Our kids never knew.) Another option is to wean your teens off cow's milk and begin using soy milk. Some researchers believe soy protein is healthier for teens than cow's milk protein.

7. Watch Your Teens' Portion Size

There's no doubt teens can eat—and eat and eat. Teens love to eat second and third helpings, and parents enjoy watching their teens enjoy eating.

There's nothing wrong with teens having a second helping, but if you put less food on their plate the first time around, they'll be ingesting fewer calories and fat grams. Try this: when they ask for a second helping of lasagna, put a smaller portion on their plates and fill the rest with salad and vegetables.

8. Do Everything You Can to Have Sit-down Dinners Together

Teens eat better when Mom or Dad is cooking and serving the food. Left to their own devices, teens would subsist on a diet of frozen pizza or microwaved chicken fingers. Yet, experts tell us that making family meals a priority is well worth the effort. A Harvard Medical School study of 16,000 children found that those who ate dinner more often with their parents had better diets.

There's no doubt the sacrosanct "Dinner Hour" is on the skids. Sure, it's sometimes impossible for everyone to eat together due to work and after-school sports schedules. The rising ranks of moms employed outside the home has greatly curtailed their enthusiasm for cooking a delicious meal. Yet eating together has a remarkable impact on the family. Of all the interventions you could pick to reduce risky behavior among teens, eating as a family is right up there. It's associated with a whole slew of positive things—and the more a family is eating together, the more positive the outcome.

A study published in the American Psychological Society newsletter found that teens who ate with their families five times or more a week were less likely to do drugs or be depressed, were more motivated at school, and had better peer relationships. A survey of National Merit scholars from the past twenty years found that, without exception, these amazing students came from families who ate together three or more nights a week. Not only can family meals make your teens smarter, but spending quality mealtimes together contributes to their emotional and spiritual growth.

I think the healthiest thing that happens during family mealtimes is communication. I loved hearing Kate and Scott ramble on about how their day went. Some of our funniest and most precious moments as a family took place around a dinner table, which is why I encourage you to make dinner together a priority—even if you have to wait until 8:00 p.m. for one of your teens to get home from football practice. (Those who are hungry can eat a healthy snack to tide them over.)

FYI... ◀◀ ▶ ❚❚ ■ ▶▶

► Great family meals don't just happen by accident. The following tried-and-true guidelines from the Larimore home will help create mealtimes everyone will cherish.

❖ Prepare the meal together. So few parents ask their teens to help out in the kitchen—and then we're surprised when they leave for college and don't even know how to boil water! Barb asked Kate and Scott to peel potatoes and carrots and to prepare salads. We learned something interesting in the process: kids involved in the cooking are more likely to eat the results!

❖ Leave the television off during meals. Our family had fallen into the bad habit of eating dinner while watching the news or some silly program. The TV is a strong competitor—you can't talk to each other, and when you're not talking to each other, you're not interacting as a family.

❖ Let the phone ring. Let the answering machine record a message.

❖ Resist the urge to go into lecture mode during mealtimes. Make mealtimes a memory, not a drudgery. Sure, you can impart wisdom in your conversing, but a family meal isn't the time to harp on what your teens are doing wrong. Keep positive communication flowing.

❖ Let your teens help in the cleanup. It rarely takes more than fifteen or twenty minutes to wash the dishes and scrub the pots and pans—even less if you have a dishwasher. It's a great habit to instill while your teens are still at home and a wonderful family activity.

A PYRAMID FOR NUTRITIONAL HEALTH

In the 1990s, the U.S. Department of Agriculture developed a food pyramid as an easy-to-follow guide to healthy eating. Food scientists at the USDA are now evaluating and revising their old pyramid, and the new one should be ready for publication by 2005. The USDA's intent was to encourage Americans to eat a more balanced diet, but many researchers and medical professionals—

myself included—believe the food pyramid relies too heavily on animal foods and refined grains and puts too little emphasis on heart-healthy fruits and vegetables. In response, a number of professionals have developed their own versions of the food pyramid. I believe Harvard researchers have come closest to getting it right, and I've adapted their pyramid ideas into my own recommendations.

Here are the building blocks of nutritional health I believe will help you encourage a lifetime of good eating habits for your teen. Don't forget: the lower levels of the pyramid are the most important!

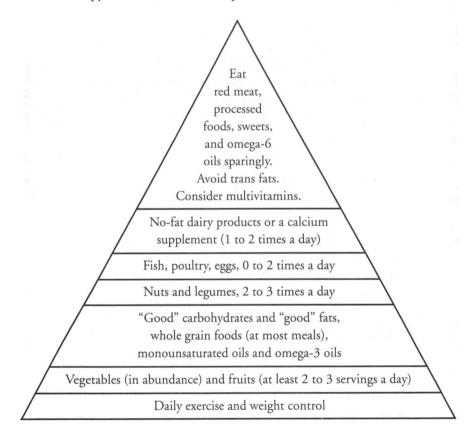

Eat
red meat,
processed
foods, sweets,
and omega-6
oils sparingly.
Avoid trans fats.
Consider multivitamins.

No-fat dairy products or a calcium
supplement (1 to 2 times a day)

Fish, poultry, eggs, 0 to 2 times a day

Nuts and legumes, 2 to 3 times a day

"Good" carbohydrates and "good" fats,
whole grain foods (at most meals),
monounsaturated oils and omega-3 oils

Vegetables (in abundance) and fruits (at least 2 to 3 servings a day)

Daily exercise and weight control

Level 1: Exercise and Weight Control

Many of the chronic diseases—such as heart attacks, strokes, diabetes, and heart disease—that plague American adults (and increasingly teens) are a direct result of obesity and inactivity. The bottom line is that it won't matter how well our teens eat if they don't get moving! When it comes to exercise, however, it can be a vicious cycle for obese and overweight teens. Because of their excessive weight, their joints hurt. Back and leg pains are their constant companions. Because their bodies ache, they don't feel like exercising, and because they can't—or won't—exercise, their body pains get worse!

Level 2: Vegetables and Fruit

Vegetables and fruits provide essential vitamins, minerals, fiber, and disease-preventing phytochemicals. Research points out the benefits of choosing leafy greens and berries. When making choices, aim for a maximum of color diversity. Every color of fruit or vegetable delivers unique health benefits.

Although five servings a day of fruits and vegetables is the standard recommendation, the more you and your teens eat the better. Some researchers now recommend up to nine servings a day for adolescent and adult men (especially African-Americans) and up to seven servings a day for adolescent and adult women to reduce the risk of cancer and other age-related diseases.

Level 3: Good Carbohydrates and Good Fats

While I explained earlier about bad carbohydrates and bad fats, some of our essential foods are good carbohydrates and good fats. No nutritional health plan is complete without them. Here's why: Whole-grain foods such as whole wheat, brown rice, and oatmeal are good sources of fiber, minerals, and some vitamins. Stone-ground whole grains are found at most grocery stores. These good carbohydrates are high in fiber and are digested more slowly, which causes a slower release of carbohydrates into the bloodstream and keeps insulin levels from reaching harmful limits.

The good fats found in certain vegetable oils, nuts, fish oil, and many plant foods also deserve a prominent place in your teen's diet. Teens who seem healthy today, if they don't consume enough good fats, can develop heart problems later in life. These monounsaturated oils (such as olive and canola oils) and omega-3 polyunsaturated fats (found in fish, canola, flax, and unhydrogenated soy oils) are considered "heart healthy" because they slow the progression of heart disease and do not raise blood cholesterol levels. The benefit of good fats is supported by evidence from Mediterranean and Nordic cultures, where people consume high amounts of these plant oils and fatty fish, yet have much lower rates of obesity, diabetes, and heart disease than Americans.

Level 4: Nuts and Legumes

Nuts provide high-quality protein and come packed with good fats. Even peanut butter—as long as it doesn't contain trans fat—is a healthy food source. Small amounts of nuts (or other foods containing good fats) actually help reduce the low-density cholesterol (LDL, or the lethal cholesterol).

Legumes are another good source of protein. The fiber in legumes helps control the appetite. Furthermore, studies indicate legumes may reduce the risk of heart disease and even prevent some forms of cancer.

Level 5: Fish, Poultry, and Eggs

Unlike red meat, fish has almost no artery-clogging saturated fat and has a healthy dose of good fats. These fats, including the omega-3 fatty acids, help make important hormones that regulate body functions. Meats that are low in saturated fats, such as poultry (chicken and turkey) without the skin, can add protein to your teen's diet with a minimum of bad fat. Eggs are also considered an excellent source of protein for teens. The latest research shows that an egg or two a day is not bad for your teen's health, so scramble some eggs in the morning. We now know that egg yolks contain two powerful phytochemicals (lutein and zeanxanthin) that promote eye health.

Level 6: Dairy Products or Calcium Supplements

A growing group of nutrition scientists believe it's unnecessary to rely on dairy foods for calcium or protein for a teen. According to research by Katherine Tucker of Tufts University, if we focused more on whole foods, such as whole grains, legumes, and fresh produce, we would create a positive mineral balance and easily meet our teen's daily calcium needs. Other good sources of calcium are low-fat yogurt, soy-based products, and calcium-fortified orange juice.

Despite the ease with which calcium needs can be met, the American Academy of Pediatrics warns that adolescents in the United States aren't getting enough calcium. Thus, the Academy recommends a daily diet that includes milk, yogurt, cheese, and other calcium-rich foods for teens. These pediatricians stress, however, that fat-reduced or fat-free dairy products are fine for older children and teens. Adolescents who cannot or will not consume adequate amounts of calcium from dietary sources should consider the use of mineral supplements.

Level 7: Eat Certain Foods Sparingly and Consider Multivitamins

Red meat, butter, white rice, white bread, potatoes, pasta, fried foods, and most sweets are placed at the top of the pyramid for a good reason—they should be eaten sparingly. Most snack foods fall into this category as well.

Most experts believe a daily multivitamin is unnecessary for teens who have a healthy diet, but how many teens eat healthy these days? Most would agree that a good daily multivitamin is not harmful to teens, and teens who have a poor diet or a chronic disease may need supplements. Keep in mind, though, that teens who pop vitamins into their mouths just so they can eat all the junk food they want are encouraging poor eating and nutrition habits.

Regardless of what you read out there, you'll never go wrong if you feed your teens a diet high in fruits, vegetables, and whole-grain foods; give them much less red meat and more fish; choose no-fat dairy foods (if you're including dairy in their diet); and choose vegetable oils and spreads rather than animal fats such as butter.

The approach you take to your teen's nutrition not only is essential to his or her health today but will dramatically affect whether he or she becomes a highly healthy young adult. Proper nutrition and exercise are areas where most parents can take practical steps to improve the balance in their teen's physical wheel.

THE LATEST TEEN TREND: GASTRIC BYPASS SURGERY

Perhaps you've heard about gastric bypass surgery, a procedure in which a bariatric surgeon "staples" the stomach—or binds it with an adjustable band—to restrict the amount of food the body can digest at one time. The surgeon creates a small pouch big enough to hold two or three ounces of food—about 10 percent of what a normal adult stomach can digest at one time. The idea is to produce a situation where it won't take long for someone to feel full when eating. Eat more, and you become nauseous and want to vomit.

Gastric bypass surgery is generally reserved for morbidly obese individuals—those with BMIs over 40 and weighing at least a hundred pounds over their normal body weight; it is now considered the treatment of choice for morbidly obese diabetics. This surgery has become incredibly popular in the last ten years as surgical techniques have improved.

The rising numbers of both obese people and surgeons who are qualified to perform these "stomach stapling" procedures has created a perfect storm in the medical world. The number of bypass operations exploded from 23,100 in 1997 to 63,100 in 2002, according to the American Society of Bariatric Surgery. Many of the leading hospitals for bypass surgery have yearlong waiting lists.

Celebrities who have gone under the knife for gastric bypass have fueled interest in the procedure. *Today* show weatherman Al Roker looks great after shedding more than a hundred pounds. Sharon Osbourne—married to wacky British rocker Ozzy Osbourne and star of the MTV reality show "The Osbournes"—said she loves to eat so much she'd probably weigh 500 pounds if she hadn't had her stomach stapled. She weighs around 130 pounds today.

I'm glad gastric bypass has worked for them, but it concerns me that some bariatric surgeons have opened their operating bay doors to teens as young as thirteen years of age. They see it as intervention—preventing obese kids from developing diabetes, joint damage, and heart disease later in life—but I worry about the options for a teen if he or she doesn't lose weight or later gains back everything he or she lost. Stapling the stomach is a surgery of no return. What can they do then?

I'm also concerned about the risk of side effects and complications. As a result of this surgery, food bypasses certain key parts of the small intestine and therefore can interfere with the absorption of essential nutrients needed by young bodies. Another potential negative side effect is "dumping syndrome"—an uncomfortable wave of nausea and an icky feeling of lightheadedness, followed by explosive diarrhea. Then there's the ultimate side effect—death. Gastric bypass has a mortality rate of between .5 and 1 percent, which means that patients have about a one in 150 chance of not surviving the surgery. Those odds wouldn't be good enough for me if I were a parent looking at all the options for my obese teen.

Gastric bypass surgery should be the surgery of last resort. I think obese teens still have time to turn around their lives by undergoing radical lifestyle changes in how much and what they eat and by adopting an exercise program. Obesity is a complicated issue, but incapacitating 90 percent of a teen's stomach is not the answer.

DYING TO BE THIN

Nor is the answer starving yourself, but that's what millions of young women with eating disorders are doing. I say "young women" because the U.S. Center for Mental Health Services estimates that more than 90 percent of those with eating disorders are females between the ages of twelve and twenty-five. Eating disorders—anorexia nervosa, bulimia nervosa, and binge-eating disorder—are a widespread problem that seems to be getting worse. In 1983, half a million young women battled anorexia. By 1998, that number had risen to more than two million. In 2001, eight million people were reported to be suffering from eating disorders.

There are important distinctions between anorexia, bulimia, and binge-eating disorder. Those with anorexia nervosa will do anything in their power *not* to eat or to eat just the bare minimum for survival. They pick at their food, leave much of it on the plate, and rigidly count calories. Those with bulimia nervosa *love* to eat, and given half the chance, they will pig out. "Biters' remorse" immediately sets in, however, and they rush to the bathroom so they can make themselves vomit the food stewing within their digestive systems. Those with binge-eating disorder go through frequent episodes of compulsive overeating, but unlike those with bulimia, they do not purge their bodies of food. Instead, they often feel shame and guilt. I've heard of girls eating a half gallon of Ben & Jerry's Cherry Garcia while their parents were out one night, and then doing a hundred push-ups and a hundred sit-ups to cancel out their high-calorie binge.

LISTEN UP!

Thin has been in for a long time, and teen girls are heavily influenced by the fashion magazines they read and the TV shows they watch. Today's supermodels must resemble a street pole to walk the runways of Milan and Paris, and TV stars like Calista Flockhart of Fox's Ally McBeal *received flattering attention for shrinking from a size 2 to an unfathomable size 0 a couple of years ago. Boyfriends can also place pressure on young women with snide comments about "thunder thighs" or "a big butt."*

Dr. Walt Larimore

Teens are especially vulnerable to developing a distorted view of themselves, which can lead to an exceedingly low self-image. If a parent, relative, or friend calls them chubby or pudgy—or refers to them as fat—they are convinced they have to lose even more weight, even if their weight is in the normal range. They come to believe the only way they can measure up is by slimming down. Eating disorders are especially common among (though certainly not limited to) young white girls who feel they need more control over their lives. Most of my anorexic patients were hyper-achievers—fashion models, dancers, and gymnasts.

Parents need to know that anorexia, bulimia, and binge eating have a severe impact on the health of teens—and can even kill them. Anorexia slows the heart rate and lowers blood pressure, increasing the chance of heart failure. Hair falls out in clumps, and nails grow brittle, as do bones. Some develop a covering of soft hair called lanugo. Those who induce vomiting wear down the enamel layer of their teeth, inflame the esophagus, and enlarge the glands near the cheeks. Peptic ulcers and long-term constipation are also consequences of bulimia. Binge eaters develop high blood pressure and high cholesterol levels and are candidates for type 2 diabetes, gallbladder disease, and heart disease.

Physiologically, the body is deprived of nutrients, so it looks elsewhere. The body begins feeding on protein in the muscles—even the heart muscle. When this happens the heart weakens, causing irregular heart rhythms and even heart failure. This is the tragic story of Karen Carpenter in a nutshell. Karen was part of a brother-sister duo known as "The Carpenters" who sang catchy tunes like "We've Only Just Begun" and "Close to You" in the 1970s and early 1980s. She wasn't overweight at all—somewhere around 120 pounds for her five-feet four-inch body, but in her mind, she could never be thin enough. So she ate and purged, ate and purged—to the point where her weight fell to 80 pounds. After collapsing on stage, she was rushed to the hospital and appeared to be making a comeback when she suddenly died of cardiac arrest at the age of thirty-two. What a tragedy!

Karen Carpenter had supposedly heard a reviewer call her chubby, and that offhand comment sent her down a highly unhealthy path. Parents seeking to nurture highly healthy teens must be careful in what they say to their teens. Don't make cutting remarks about their weight or tease them about how puberty has them "packing a few more pounds." If you're on a diet, don't constantly talk about it at the dinner table. Continue to serve three well-balanced meals a day. Remind your teen often that they are beautiful creatures of God.

Finally, watch for telltale signs, such as frequent visits to the bathroom, watery eyes from gagging, and music playing in the bathroom to muffle purging sounds. Bags of snacks and ice cream cartons that disappear overnight should raise suspicions.

I've often talked with parents of girls with eating disorders who realized later that their daughters left behind a rabbit trail of clues—obsessing about the fat grams in a slice of pizza, wondering how many calories were in a home-made chocolate chip cookie, searching the refrigerator for the salad dressing with the least amount of fat, picking at their food and leaving two-thirds of the meal uneaten, and panicking when the scale said they weighed one pound more than they weighed last week. (Please note that a teen girl who *occasionally* exhibits this behavior doesn't necessarily have a problem, but if the pattern persists, it's something you'll want to keep an eye on.)

Parents, if you sense your teen daughter or son may have an eating disorder, get help *now*! You are dealing with a potentially fatal situation. It's best not to confront your teen until you learn more about the best treatment options. Your family doctor is a good place to start.

Check It Out!

▶ I highly recommend psychiatric intervention for those with eating disorders, and I remember many times when I authorized a hospitalization. Teens don't develop an eating disorder overnight, and they won't get well overnight. You may have to consider a residential facility, and two of the best in the nation, in my opinion, are the Remuda Ranch in Wickenburg, Arizona, and the Meier Clinic Day Hospital in Dallas, Texas. You can learn more on my website (www.highlyhealthy.net).

Eating disorders are tied into teens' self-image, and during the adolescent years, the way they look means everything to these youngsters. I'll discuss why physical appearance is so important to teens in our next chapter, as well as what parents can do about the rising popularity of tattoos and other forms of "body art."

Chapter 7

FOR APPEARANCE' SAKE

When Scott was twelve or thirteen, we were sitting on a dock one afternoon, kicking at the water with our bare feet. A black cloud seemed to be hanging over Scott. "What are you thinking about?" I asked cheerfully, hoping to brighten his dark mood.

He hung his head and whispered, "I'm ugly."

I pondered his statement for a moment. "Who told you that?"

"All I have to do is look in the mirror, and I know I'm ugly."

My parental assessment was shaken. Scott was a cute blond-haired, blue-eyed kid who wasn't overweight and didn't have acne. Yet he still thought he was ugly.

I came to realize he was doing what many adolescents do—comparing himself to other kids. Comparing himself to glossy, airbrushed images of celebrities in popular magazines. Comparing himself to images he saw on television and in movies. Coming to the wrong conclusions!

Parents seeking to nurture highly healthy adolescents need to understand that peer pressure and media pressure can squash their spirits like a steamroller crushing a pop can. You need to be the voice of reason in their lives, reminding them that true beauty is more than bulging biceps and hourglass figures, more than having the right eye color or wearing a certain hairstyle. Barb and I didn't spend much time complimenting external things like new outfits or jewelry; instead, we chose to compliment Scott's infectious laughter or gave Kate "attagirl's" for her remarkable ability to read books quickly or memorize Bible verses.

That afternoon on the dock with Scott, I remember sharing 1 Samuel 16:7, the verse where God spoke to Samuel about whom he should pick to be his successor to the throne:

> But the LORD said to Samuel, "Do not consider his appearance or his height, for I have rejected him. The LORD does not look at the things man looks at. Man looks at the outward appearance, but the LORD looks at the heart."

I reminded Scott that God doesn't consider physical appearance to be important, so why should we? God is more interested in our character than our appearance, I told him. "Scott, the average person doesn't look like a model on a magazine cover. In fact, the average model does *not* look that good in real life because of all the retouching they do to photos. God had it right: the heart is more important."

Scott grunted his agreement, but it was a hard concept to accept at his age. During adolescence, boys and girls undergo rapid changes, especially in their looks. Teens, as they awaken to the world around them, spend hours in front of the mirror fussing with their hair or scanning their faces for blemishes. They are obsessed with the way they look to others. Their greatest desire is to fit in. The last thing they want is to be teased by schoolmates for any imperfection—perceived or otherwise!

Then one day Scott came with a request to let his buddies highlight his hair. Several friends had colored their hair, he said, so it was the in thing to do. Since those blond streaks would modify his appearance, Scott knew he needed permission from Barb and me first.

Back then, Scott sported a thatch of to-die-for blond hair. Although Barb and I thought he needed highlighted hair like Britney Spears needed another pair of hip-hugging jeans, we gave him our blessing. We made it clear, however, that he would have to live with the consequences of the results. What if his hair turned out to have green or blue spikes? That happens sometimes when kids are mixing chemicals.

As to the fundamental issue of whether Scott could highlight his hair, Barb and I had resolved not to make a big deal about it. In our minds, hair was hair—one of the body's renewable resources that grows back after being cut, colored, or curled. Since we were sure Scott had asked to highlight his hair because his friends were doing it, we used his hair-coloring request as a parental opportunity to let the tether line out a little further. In the greater scheme of push-pull issues between parents and children, hair coloring wasn't worth going to the ramparts for.

I did have some questions for Scott, however:

- ❖ Why do you want to highlight your hair? Is it a fad? Are you doing it simply to fit in?
- ❖ Do you know any mature Christian men—pastors, elders, Christian leaders—who highlight their hair? If not, why do you think that is?
- ❖ Have you prayed about it? If so, what is God telling you?
- ❖ How will having highlighted hair affect your witness for God?

We had a great discussion that evening at dinner. After our family talked it through, with everyone having a say, he decided, with our blessing, to think about it a bit more.

So what happened after Scott kicked it around his mind? He decided to take a pass. I think what happened is that after he and his buddies highlighted his friend Kyle's hair, he lost interest in the stunt.

Barb and I handled Scott's hair highlighting episode by asking ourselves five questions—ones you can employ whenever your teens want to do something you consider off the wall. (You'll find our incident-specific answers in italics.)

1. Is what he is asking to do illegal?
   No. As far as we knew, Lady Clairol was not contraband.

2. Is he going to hurt himself?
   No, although he may break a few hearts among his young female friends.

3. Is it going to make a difference in five years?
   No. Highlights have a shelf life of a month or two.

4. Is it something that will hurt someone else?
   No. But his friends better wear gloves and a mask when applying that nasty-smelling stuff.

5. Is it inappropriate for his age?
   No. It's exactly the type of crazy antics teens do.

Since we couldn't answer yes to any of those questions, we were led to approve his request. We believed that any activity (such as hair highlighting or getting an earring) not discussed in the Bible was just a different choice, not necessarily a wrong choice—unless the motive was wrong. Now, I understand that some parents may approach this situation differently, but for us, it wasn't a battle worth fighting.

If Scott had wanted to get a Mohawk, we probably would have opposed it. While he wasn't asking to do anything illegal, it could have hurt him because kids with Mohawks were treated like pariahs in our small town. And to be honest, he would have embarrassed Barb and me because shaving his sidewalls and leaving a swatch of hair on the crown of his head would have been out of the mainstream with the families we hung out with. We would have discussed with him the reasons we wouldn't allow him to get a Mohawk and outlined the consequences of disobedience.

A BRANDING MOMENT

Thankfully, Scott never pressed us to get a Mohawk haircut. During his freshman year of college, however, he raised the topic of tattoos, wondering out loud if he should get one someday. In some ways, I didn't blame him—"tats" were everywhere, and some of his dorm buddies sported them. They've become very popular in our culture. There may not be a Hollywood entertainer or music artist under the age of thirty who doesn't have a tattoo on some part of his or her body. According to a Harris Interactive poll, around 16 percent of adult Americans have at least one tattoo, believing that body art makes them feel sexier, more rebellious, and even more intelligent.

Scott never asked our permission to get a tattoo, but we could tell he was seriously thinking about it after one of his friends got one between his shoulder blades. To Barb and me, a tattoo was several floors up from coloring his hair. Part of it was cultural—the only people who had tattoos in the sixties were the circus's bearded lady, leather-clad bikers on their Harley Davidsons, and square-jawed Marines.

So Barb and I asked ourselves the five questions:

1. Is what he is asking to do illegal?
   No. Because Scott has turned eighteen, he can legally get a tattoo.

2. Is he going to hurt himself?
   Possibly. Tattoo parlors are unregulated, and many are unsanitary and undependable. Those on the sharp end of a tattoo needle risk infection for everything from hepatitis B to HIV. I've seen evidence that the blood from a previous customer can contaminate the line carrying the ink to the needle.

3. Is it going to make a difference in five years?

Yes. Tattoos are permanent. Yes, they can be surgically removed by laser, or a plastic surgeon can cauterize the skin—burning it off and replacing the area with skin grafts—but it's excruciatingly painful. Plus, tattoo removal is expensive. Insurance companies put it in the same category as plastic surgery—an elective they won't cover. We're talking thousands of out-of-pocket dollars.

4. Is it something that will hurt someone else?
   Frankly, both Barb and I would have felt hurt if Scott had gone ahead and gotten a tattoo. Finally, a point worth making is that a tattoo may have hurt Scott's job prospects in the future.

5. Is it inappropriate for his age?
   Yes, in our opinion. Scott was just starting adult life, and that tattoo would be on his body for the rest of his life.

FYI . . .   ◀◀ ▶ ❚❚ ■ ▶▶

► *What about "Temporary" Tattoos?*

If your teen is clamoring for a "temporary" tattoo, be sure to tell him or her about the dangers of black henna tattoos, which are advertised to last less than a month but may leave a lifetime of scars and horrible blisters. Tattoo artists are using a form of black henna (an ink) that has been mixed with commercial hair dye, which includes a chemical called p-phenylenediamine, or PPD. PPD gives the tattoo ink its coal tar color, but this ingredient causes allergic reactions in some people. While this may sound benign, what I've read is that teens are noticing burn marks on their skin as the tattoo fades. Others develop swelling or severe rashes that ooze. Bottom line: there may be nothing temporary about "temporary" tattoos.

Talking Tattoos with Your Teen

Because tattoos are so popular these days, and because impulsive teens walking down the boardwalk may step into a tattoo parlor, I'd be proactive and talk to your teen right away about how you feel. If you wait too long, he or she might come home with your worst nightmare indelibly inked on their skin.

Here are some points to emphasize:

❖ *God created our bodies.* If the body is a temple of the Holy Spirit, as the New Testament teaches (1 Corinthians 6:19), then painting permanent graffiti on the temple walls may not be practicing the best stewardship.

❖ *Consider how long the tattoo will be on the skin.* Take the story of actor and rockabilly singer Billy Bob Thornton, who had "Angelina" tattooed on his left forearm after he married movie star Angelina Jolie. She matched his commitment, having "Billy Bob" scripted in black ink high on her left arm. Yet, when the marriage broke up, guess what happened? The tattooed names were still there—which produced an interesting "solution." Billy Bob covered his former wife's name with a new angel tattoo, while Angelina underwent painful laser surgery to remove "Billy Bob" from her left arm.

The problem goes beyond inking someone's name on your skin. Other kinds of tattoos—barbed wire, Chinese characters, soaring eagles, tribal feathers, rose petals, or even Christian symbols—become dated as they fall out of fashion. Case in point: the WWJD (What Would Jesus Do?) fad that seems to have run its course. Not many kids wear WWJD bracelets these days. Ask your teen if he thinks it'd be cool to get a WWJD tattooed to his left bicep, and he'll undoubtedly tell you it would look dorky. There's your answer.

❖ *It's expensive, painful, and time-consuming to remove tattoos.* I don't care if Angelina Jolie hired the best plastic surgeon Hollywood money can buy, she still paid a heavy price to have her "Billy Bob" tattoo removed. I've seen pictures of her left arm, and it looks as though someone used Photoshop to strip in a light rectangle of skin where the tattoo used to be. Tattoo removal is not for the squeamish. In Angelina's case, a laser vaporized the black pigment with a high-intensity light beam. Black tattoo pigment absorbs all laser wavelengths, making it the easiest to treat; other colors, such as green, selectively absorb laser light, making it tough to erase. Laser surgery is far from perfect, but it's a huge improvement over dermabrasion, where the skin is sanded to remove the surface and middle layers. Other methods include cryosurgery, which freezes the tattooed skin before removing the tattoo, and surgical excision, in which a surgeon removes the tattoo with a scalpel and closes the wound with stitches.

❖ *The risk of infection is way too high.* There are no guarantees that the electric needle has been sterilized for the next customer. I wouldn't bet my future on it, but that's what teens do every time they get tattooed. The ink line between the tank and the electric needle typically doesn't get changed between tattoos, so a person's blood cells may contaminate the line. The risk of contracting blood-borne infections, such as hepatitis B or hepatitis C, is not low, which explains why blood banks won't accept blood for at least a year after someone has received a tattoo.

❖ *Know that your teen may be able to get a tattoo without your permission.* While teens have to be adults (age eighteen) to get a tattoo in most states, fifteen states have *no* laws regarding tattooing and body piercing at any age. Some states have laws that allow tattoos and body piercing with parental consent as early as age sixteen, and only four states ban the practice outright—Massachusetts, Oklahoma, South Carolina, and Vermont. Whether it's legal or not, I wouldn't bank on tattoo parlors checking ID whenever someone wanting a tattoo appears on their doorstep with $100 cash in his or her pocket.

FYI . . . ⏪ ▶ ⏸ ⏹ ⏩

▶ *What If Your Teen Insists on Getting a Tattoo?*

You'll first want to consider whether the desire to get a tattoo is well motivated and not related to rebellion or acting out. Something in the latter category requires a completely different approach. (By the way, issues such as "getting pierced," "going to a rave," and "dating at age fourteen" could be substituted for "getting a tattoo.")

If rebellion is not the issue at hand, and you still don't approve of your teen's request, you and your spouse must decide *why* you don't approve. Is your disapproval reasonable? Since most of these kinds of issues aren't specifically addressed in the Bible, are they what the Bible calls "disputable" situations in which different Christian parents can decide differently?

Consider studying Romans 14 and linking it with Ephesians 6:4—then pray about what you learn. You may also want to discuss the issue with your pastor or other respected Christian parents. Then, if you conclude that the activity isn't appropriate, you'll want to sit down as a family and discuss your decision with your teen. This discussion should include the reasons for your decision and the consequences of disobedience.

On the other hand, if you don't approve but you're willing to allow your teen to make the decision without your full blessing, make it a point to sit down as a family and to be very honest as you discuss your feelings.

Body Art

I started noticing patients with tattoos back in the mid-1990s, when NBA basketball star Dennis Rodman received an avalanche of media attention for tattooing and piercing most of the available real estate on his six-feet eight-inch body. ESPN pundits and sports columnists lapped it up and turned him into a folk hero: the iconoclast rebounder who dyed his short Afro hair in various shades of red, white, and blue and thumbed his nose—which had a diamond stud in the left nostril—at the Establishment. Almost single-handedly, Rodman introduced "body art" to the nation's living rooms, though I have to admit I'm still not used to it.

Overnight, the entertainment industry rushed in and promoted body art—the piercing of various cartilage, skin, and orifices or the permanent coloring of skin with inks and dyes—until it became part of the mainstream. This cultural shift trickled into my examination room, where I began seeing high school teens and young adults with tattoos and a dizzying array of piercings. I'm talking about a half dozen earrings hanging on one ear, a string of eyebrow rings across the brow, and an assortment of nose rings, nose studs, lip rings, chin studs, labrets (a stud through the lower lip), and tongue studs.

Piercing is just what it sounds like—the piercing of the body with needles ranging from a 2 gauge (what a veterinarian would use on a horse) to a 20 gauge (what you're pricked with when getting a flu shot). Ears are the most common places for piercings, but the eyebrows, nose, and tongue are where the action is these days.

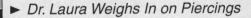

FYI . . .

► *Dr. Laura Weighs In on Piercings*

Radio talk-show host Dr. Laura Schlessinger was once in Colorado Springs and asked whether she could borrow Focus on the Family's broadcast studio to do her daily radio show. I dropped by the control booth to watch Dr. Laura in action.

I'll never forget the call Dr. Laura took from a teen girl who said she was thinking of getting her tongue pierced. "I'm pretty sure my parents won't approve, but I'm thinking about doing it behind their back," she said. "Before I did, I thought I'd call you because I respect you and your opinion."

From my perch behind the control room's plate-glass window, I thought the radio psychologist would begin by saying how destructive it was to do something behind the back of those in authority. Perhaps she'd make the point that God gave parents authority over children for a reason, so anytime a child does something to destroy the trust built in the relationship, it can't be a good thing.

Dr. Laura didn't take that tack at all. "Do you know who the speaker of the House is?" she asked.

"Dennis Hastert," the girl responded.

"Do you know who the chief justice of the U.S. Supreme Court is?"

"Rehnquist."

Dr. Laura went through a list of influential people, and the girl nailed most of them.

"How many of these people have a pierced tongue?" Dr. Laura inquired.

"Ah, none."

"Why do you think none of them do?"

She didn't have an answer for that.

"I'll bet you have friends who are piercing their tongues," Dr. Laura commented.

"Yes, I do."

"Isn't that why you want to do it?"

"Well, yeah."

"Are your friends the type of people growing up to be the type of person you want to be? If the answer is no, then you have some decisions to make—important decisions that will affect your future. I won't tell you what those decisions should be, but I think you know in your heart what you need to do."

"I think I know what I need to do," the teen said.

"I think you do too."

What was interesting was what the listening audience couldn't see. During the commercial break, I saw Dr. Laura with a big smile on her face. She licked her pointer finger and made a line in the air—toting one up for the good guys. If you've nurtured your teens right—keeping the right amount of air in all their wheels—you'll be able to tote them up as good guys too.

Many young people pierce themselves or have a friend stick a safety pin into their bodies to form the hole, which is medically unsound at best and incredibly stupid at worst. For instance, a friend will pinch her friend's right eyebrow, jab the safety pin, work the pin through the skin and muscle, and then remove the safety pin and insert a lightweight hoop ring. I doubt one in a thousand are aware that they could sever a nerve in the eyebrow that controls the eye muscles.

Oral piercings are bad news. The American Dental Association opposes piercing of the tongue, lip, and cheek, calling it a public health hazard. The American Academy of Dermatology takes it one step further: they oppose all forms of body piercing with one exception—the earlobe. Unlike other areas of the body, earlobes are made up of fatty tissue and have a strong blood supply.

Pierced teens open themselves up to infection, scarring, tetanus (which can be fatal), boils (or infections under the skin), permanent holes or deforming scars in the nose or eyebrow, and chipped or broken teeth from biting on a tongue stud. Some develop a speech impediment because of tongue studs in their mouths.

As I've done physicals over the years, I've noted piercings in some unimaginable places: the nipples, the navel, and—I'm not making this up—the genitalia. Dennis Rodman told the media he had his scrotum pierced, but that's nothing compared to the "Prince Albert"—the insertion of a needle-receiving tube into the urethra. The Prince Albert ring goes into and along the male urethra and comes out behind the glans on the underside of the penis. Girls are piercing themselves south of the border as well—having their labia majora pierced with rings.

Why Would Your Teen Pierce?

In my opinion, many teens are experiencing a crisis of confidence that penetrates deep into their hearts. Teen girls want to know that their parents think they are lovely and worthy of their attention and affection. Teen boys want to know—especially from their fathers—that they have what it takes, that their dads admire them and consider them special. Sadly, many teens are growing up believing they are unloved by their parents. A subset of these teens also thinks they are hated or disrespected by their peers. This lack of affirmation and unconditional love can result in a low self-image at best and a self-loathing or self-hatred at worst.

Whenever I saw piercings or tattoos in my practice, I'd make a mental note that this could be a teen at risk. Why? Low self-esteem and self-loathing can serve as a prelude to severely harmful behavior such as violence, drug abuse, promiscuity, and suicide. Of course, not all piercings or tattoos represent psychological, relational, or spiritual disorders. Teens may do it just for the attention or because their friends are doing it. They may do it to get a rise out of Mom and Dad. Or it may represent an attempt to demonstrate independence or be the result of peer pressure.

For most teens, however, the failure to feel affirmed and loved helps explain why they do things that would otherwise make no sense—piercing sensitive body parts; tattooing themselves from head to toe; cutting their flesh; taking dangerous drugs; and identifying themselves with death, perversion, and satanic ritual.

BEYOND THE FRINGE

Rebellious teens may search for something *more* to rebel against as "tats" and piercings become more accepted (and even considered "normal"). This kind of thinking is leading down the path to tongue splitting, toe shortening, and other forms of self-injury. These things may sound bizarre to our ears, but I don't think any generation can predict what the next one will rebel against.

Tongue Splitting

I don't believe tongue splitting is destined to catch on, but I would have said the same thing about the Prince Albert. In "forking" the tongue, a medically untrained "technician" slices the median fibrous septum that centrally divides the tongue right down the middle—usually wielding a previously used surgical blade or a knife that has been heated over a flame. It gives me shivers just thinking about it!

We have no long-term data on the impact of tongue splitting. Nor do we have any evidence that the procedure is reversible. I can only imagine that it's incredibly painful to undergo because the tongue has gazillions of sensitive nerves. To me, it appears to be another sign of teens crying out for help.

Toe Shortening

Fashion-hungry young women are having the tips of their toes surgically scaled back so they can squeeze their feet into pointy shoes made popular on shows like *Sex and the City*. Adolescents or young adults who go to such extremes for attention may suffer from psychological issues. If the activity involves something that hurts or changes your body, there's typically a self-esteem problem. The more you see this kind of behavior, the less likely it is that the teen can be called highly healthy.

Self-Injury

Self-injury (cutting, or self-mutilation or self-abuse) is another example of highly unhealthy behavior. Teens who cut often take a razor blade or Exacto knife to slice their legs, arms, wrists, and ribs. Those who cut say they experience a great relieving of stress when they dig into the skin and start themselves bleeding. To them, the stress reduction is similar to the way a teakettle lets off steam when the water is boiling. Cutting gives teens a sense of power and a feeling of being able to control the emotional pain in their lives.

It would seem that parents would have to be sleepwalking not to notice the telltale scars on their teens' legs, wrists, and arms—or the bloody tissues in the garbage bag—but teens usually go out of their way to shield their behavior. I heard about a Florida teen who began cutting herself after nicking her leg with a razor while taking a shower. The release of blood felt good, she said, so she cut herself again. In her mind, it was pain releasing pain. But then she became unable to stop, cutting her forearms, wrists, and ribs nearly every day. To cover up her handiwork, she wore a sweatshirt year-round. (Believe me, that's hard to do in Florida!) She hid bloodstained towels in her closet and washed them when her parents were away.

Called the "new age anorexia," the practice of self-mutilating behavior is said to be on the rise. It is estimated that one out of every 200 teen girls in the U.S. between the ages of thirteen and nineteen regularly practices self-abusive behavior. A British study of over 6,000 pupils (ages fifteen and sixteen), conducted by the Centre for Suicide Research at Oxford University, revealed that more than one teen out of ten deliberately harmed themselves, with nearly two-thirds from cutting. Teens with low self-esteem, anxiety, or depression—those who shut themselves in their room rather than talk things through—were more likely to hurt themselves.

It's very difficult in a high school assembly full of teens to identify a person who practices self-abusive behaviors. He or she is generally a good student, has a normal or above-normal appearance, is involved in school and after-school activities, and has parents who are involved in the community. The parents, however, often aren't highly involved in their teen's life. In many cases, both parents work outside the home and have above-average income levels. Often a self-abusive teen will avoid activities that require changing clothes at school, since he or she wants to keep the self-harmful behavior a secret—which may explain why many tend not to have close friends.

Self-mutilating teens often internalize any conflicts with friends, schoolmates, or parents because they don't want to "cause trouble" for anyone. The fear, anxiety, isolation, and emotional pain inside can build to a point where these teens feel they might explode. To prevent this explosion—and to deal with the emotions they're feeling—they cut or burn or pick in an attempt to bleed them out. It's their form of release and becomes a coping mechanism; it's how they deal with life and everything it offers. Some of these adolescents also have suicidal thoughts or would accept death as one possible consequence of self-harm, but this is only true for a minority.

Girls have a higher prevalence of self-harm, up to four times more than boys. Experts believe that self-aggressive behavior of girls may be related to sexual abuse, while self-aggressive boys may have suffered physical abuse. Contrary to popular opinion, these adolescents are typically not just seeking attention or trying to frighten someone.

LISTEN UP!

Cutting, or self-mutilation, is a flashing warning light of poor self-esteem, a clear signal that something painful is bottled up inside. Do not attempt to fix this problem alone; you need professional help. A family physician is a great place to start because he or she can coordinate the proper mental health care your teen needs at this crossroads moment in his or her life. Ask your family physician to recommend a good Christian psychologist or psychiatrist.

Dr. Walt Larimore

WE MUST, WE MUST INCREASE OUR . . .

Anne Weisman's play *Be Aggressive* is a dark comedy about a cheerleader from one of the snazzier zip codes in Southern California who can't wait for her high school graduation present from her parents—breast implants.

We laugh because it sounds preposterous, but it's happening. Cosmetic surgery is the rage these days, and the frequency of teens seeking some form of plastic surgery—breast augmentation, rhinoplasty (a nose job), or otoplasty (the pinning back of protruding ears)—is growing by the day.

Each year, 3 percent of those eighteen and younger undergo cosmetic procedures, according to the American Society of Plastic Surgeons. While it may not sound like a large number, three out of every hundred teen girls submitting to elective cosmetic surgery each year is surely a lot higher than it used to be. Since the late 1990s, the number of teen girls having breast augmentation has quadrupled, and the tally for liposuction has tripled. The rising numbers concern me and have triggered a debate about the appropriateness of teen cosmetic surgery.

I'm not talking about repairing a scar or fixing a nose that got broken during a football game. I can also see why an older teen girl with very large breasts might seek breast reduction surgery to alleviate shoulder pains, breathing difficulties, and embarrassment in social situations. I'm also sympathetic to someone who has had nasal trauma and was left with a disfigured nose—a bulky lump for all the world to see. But these are the exceptions, not the rule.

If I were a cosmetic surgeon, I wouldn't give my approval to most elective cosmetic surgery procedures on teens until they had undergone extensive psychological (or psychiatric) testing. Many of the young women who pursue elective surgery to have bigger breasts or their ears pinned have one or more significantly flattened wheels. Often it's the case that they have a terrible relationship with God or with their parents, or they are seeking affirmation, acceptance, and love in the wrong places. I would want to know why a young woman wanted breast augmentation before I agreed to perform the procedure.

The same goes for liposuction—a procedure in which a suction catheter is stuck underneath the skin so fat cells can be suctioned away. This invasive operation, which allows the removal of unwanted fat and some body sculpting, comes with a host of possible complications, including bruising, swelling, bleeding, infection, and change in nerve function. I can think of very few cases where liposuction would be appropriate on teen bodies that are still growing.

A couple of additional cautions: Any doctor can hang out his shingle and perform plastic surgery without having attained a specialty degree. Also be aware that plastic surgery is a lucrative business because it's cash up-front. The vast majority of cosmetic procedures are elective and not covered by private insurance. For any cosmetic surgery that is indicated and appropriate, be sure you seek at least two opinions from surgeons who are residency trained and board certified in plastic surgery.

THE RAVAGES OF ACNE

There is a form of cosmetic surgery for teens I wholeheartedly endorse—plastic surgery for those who have facial scars from severe acne. Like it or not, first impressions are lasting impressions in our society, and a teen with severe acne can feel like a modern-day version of a leper from Bible times.

Thankfully, not many cases of acne need the intervention of a plastic surgeon. But no matter how little or how much acne teens have on their faces, it's an affliction I treated fairly aggressively in my practice. Acne can be devastating to a teen's self-esteem and subject him or her to horrible comments from their peers ("Hey, pizza face!").

Acne is synonymous with adolescence and puberty (adults rarely have it—though their faces may still show scars from teen blemishes). This facial affliction usually crops up when a teen turns fourteen or fifteen years old, but I've seen kids as young as eleven or twelve with cystic acne.

Acne is an inflammatory disease of the sebaceous (oil-producing) glands, characterized by blackheads and pustules and, in severer forms, by cysts and scarring. The lesions appear on the face, but they can also crop up on the neck, shoulders, and back. Although the exact cause is unknown, acne is undoubtedly related to the increased hormonal activity that occurs during puberty.

In mild cases, simple facial cleansing twice a day works wonders. Over-the-counter products, such as Oxy 5, which contains 5 percent benzoyl peroxide, are effective as well. It was once thought that acne was caused by foods rich in carbohydrates and fat (such as chocolate and nuts), but research has negated that long-held view. The latest research shows that stress aggravates acne. The good news is that severe acne is fairly treatable these days—and the earlier it's treated, the better. The following is a typical conversation I would have in my examination room:

Me: I notice you've got some screamers there, Jim. Something you wrestle with a lot, or is it just something you get at the end of the summer?

Jim: No, I get these guys all the time, and they're terrible.

Me: Well, listen, I just want you to know there are some incredibly effective treatments available now for acne. It may not even take more than one visit to get you the help you need. We have ways of preventing these guys and teaching you how to take care of them. Sound like a plan?

Whenever I had such a conversation, I'd tell the parents that their son's or daughter's acne was an appearance issue he or she shouldn't have to wrestle with. There are so many effective treatments for acne these days. Even the most severe and scarring form of acne can now be treated and—if caught early enough—be prevented. If none of the simpler, less expensive forms of therapy work, there's a nearly miraculous drug called Accutane—a vitamin A derivative containing isotretinoin that offers a chance of curing severe acne. Accutane is a potent drug that effectively rids the skin of cystic or scarring acne. It has a remarkable 95 percent success rate when dosed correctly, and teens who have seen their skin clear up are reporting that they've stayed acne-free for ten to fifteen years. (The most difficult thing to like is Accutane's high cost—upwards of $3,000, including doctor's visits, lab tests, and medication costs. A generic version of the drug is now available, which significantly lowers the cost.)

It's important to note that Accutane should be reserved for treating the most serious forms of acne. Among its side effects are serious birth defects and fetal death for the unborn baby if the mother takes the drug while pregnant (or gets pregnant while taking the drug). Despite intense efforts to keep the drug away from pregnant women, the FDA has had over two thousand reports in the last decade of women becoming pregnant during the time they were taking Accutane. Therefore, the FDA has initiated a program that makes it far tougher for women to get the prescription drug. Accutane also has side effects that teens need to be aware of—dry mouth, dry nose, and cracked skin around the mouth. In my opinion, it's a small price to pay for having an acne-free face.

You don't necessarily need to see a dermatologist to start your teen on Accutane. Some pediatricians and family physicians are certified and experienced in overseeing Accutane treatment, which lasts for twenty to twenty-two weeks. In 2003, however, the FDA (in cooperation with the manufacturer, Roche Laboratories) began a new program called SMART (System to Manage Accutane Related Teratogenicity)—designed to enhance the safe, appropriate use of Accutane by strengthening the existing Accutane Pregnancy Prevention Program (PPP), a comprehensive patient education program. You can learn more about these programs and Accutane's risks and benefits at my website (www.highlyhealthy.net).

We covered some heavy topics in this chapter, and all the role models may seem to come from popular culture. While pop figures set trends and make fashion statements, don't underestimate for one minute the importance of being a role model to your teens. The tone you set in the home and the values you espouse are being heard by your teens—even though it might not seem like it at times. In the pages ahead, we'll talk about the importance of giving them a solid upbringing, and we'll outline the direction families are taking.

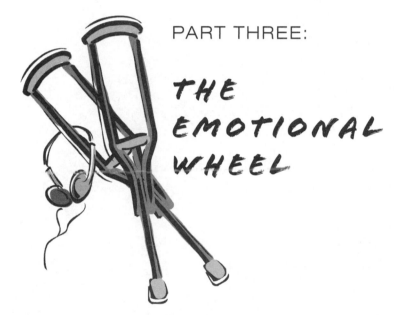

PART THREE:

THE
EMOTIONAL
WHEEL

Chapter 8

THE ABC'S—AND D'S—OF NURTURING YOUR TEEN

Highly healthy teens need four things from their parents to maintain their emotional health during their preteen and adolescent years. They're as simple as A-B-C-D:

* ❖ A = Affirmation
* ❖ B = Blameless love
* ❖ C = Connectedness
* ❖ D = Discipline

I define emotional health as the state of one's emotional and mental well-being. I know that mixing the words *teen*, *emotional*, and *mental well-being* is like mixing chili powder into a cake mix—they're disagreeable ingredients. Teens *are* highly emotional, and it's easy to question their mental well-being. Anyone who has spent time around teens has witnessed their incredible highs and the earth-shattering lows. One moment they're on top of the world ("I aced my biology test!"), and the next moment they're inconsolable ("I'm ruined—no one asked me to the homecoming bash").

There will be days when your teen's emotional wheel will be pumped to the point of bursting, and there will be days when it's flatter than a crêpe suzette. Their sudden mood shifts cause everyone to be on edge. As you might suspect, hormones are the underlying reason behind their inflated highs and out-of-air lows.

These are the times to maintain a steady hand on the rudder. Just as a sudden jerk of the wheel can tip a boat over, any emotional overreactions from your side will feel unsettling to them. Maintain an even keel and a steady course. Look for opportunities to *affirm* and approve. *Love* them unconditionally, even when they're driving you crazy. Stay *connected*, even though they're away from the house more often, and ensure that their out-of-home connections are highly healthy. Maintain *discipline* (coaching and cheerleading) as you continue to train these adolescents so they can become self-sufficient, highly healthy young adults.

I know it wasn't long ago that these teens were cuddly creatures who hung on your every word and accepted everything you said at face value. Now they're growing up and leaving childhood, beginning a journey that will take them to the Land of Adults. They're not quite there. Teens aren't mature enough or prepared enough to go it alone or to have life all figured out—and that's simply because they're still teens.

This is the time when you need to be an emotional rock for them. The teen years are a critical time for mothers to be stay-at-home moms—or at least to be home when they arrive home after the end of the school day. And it isn't a time for Dad to be AWOL either. When parents are physically present and emotionally available, they strengthen family intimacy and build healthier children.

Let's take a closer look at how the A-B-C-D acrostic relates to your teen's emotional health:

AFFIRMATION

During the teen years, affirmation and approval are crucial. Your young man wants to know, Do I have what it takes? Am I becoming a man in your eyes? Your young woman wants to know, Am I lovely? Am I precious? Am I worthy of pursuit?

You must be your child's best cheerleader. Think about it: if you're not cheering on your teen, who is? He or she needs your "way to go" and "I'm so proud of you" more than you know. Too many parents major on critique and forget to cheer.

Words carry incredible power. In her book *Living History*, Hillary Rodham Clinton noted she's never forgotten the time she brought home a straight-A report card from high school. She proudly showed it to her dad, hoping for a word of commendation. Instead, he said, "Well, you must be attending an easy school." Decades later, that offhand remark still burns in Mrs. Clinton's mind. His thoughtless response might have represented nothing more than a casual quip, but it created a point of pain that has endured to this day.

Be sure to affirm your teen in both words and deeds. I heard Michael Reagan, adopted son of former president Ronald Reagan, talk about this in a radio interview.

> We were all sent to boarding school. The Crosby kids, the Hope kids, and all of us went to boarding school. So at five and a half years old, I'd be dropped off at boarding school and come home every other weekend. That was a terrible thing for me. I was saying to myself, "Why doesn't my family want me? Why are the other kids being picked up every day and going home to eat dinner with their mothers and their dads and I'm not?" I started to feel bad about myself. I thought there was something inherently wrong with me. I began to keep secrets from my parents and not talk to them because I felt, "You didn't want to talk to me, so I'm not going to talk back."

Michael Reagan made this concluding observation: "Every child needs affirmation—male, female, it doesn't matter—we all need to be affirmed. If the parents aren't there to affirm the child, somebody else will pick up the reins and affirm that child."

Remember, if you aren't your teen's cheerleader, he or she will look for affirmation elsewhere. For a young woman, it could be the warm embrace of some guy you probably don't know. When he whispers sweet nothings in her ear, telling her that she's the most beautiful creature he's ever seen, that she's so special, we shouldn't be surprised when she becomes putty in his arms—even to the point of giving him her virginity. She wants romance and affirmation, while he wants sex. In her mind, being affirmed is worth even *that*.

A young man living without affirmation will seek it elsewhere too—usually from other guys. Teens looking for affirmation can find it, in its worst manifestation, in gangs that search for willing recruits in all shapes and sizes. Gangs are equal opportunity employers, drawing in disenfranchised kids and reaching into middle-class neighborhoods. Boys from single-parent households are especially vulnerable because they're seeking the male approval they're not currently experiencing.

Young males craving affirmation can also find it from a group of guys—a "set" or a "posse"—who aren't selling drugs, painting graffiti, or settling turf battles. This group of guys chooses to hang out together (usually at a friend's house whose parents are never home) because they receive approval and affirmation from each other. These kids sometimes get into drugs or drinking, but they could also be drawn to each other by a mutual fascination for violent video games. If your teen boy is asking to hang out with his friends every free moment, that's a good sign he's finding love and affirmation more outside than inside your home.

It takes time, effort, and opportunity to be your teen's cheerleader. You have to take the moments as they come. I witnessed such a moment not long ago when I walked through a large department store with Barb. She was shopping, and I was people watching—one of my favorite hobbies. I saw a tall, gangly African-American teen boy walking behind a woman I assumed was his mom. "Adrian," I overheard her say, "when you grow up you'll make a fantastic husband for some very lucky young woman. I'm *so* proud of what you are becoming."

She kept walking and talking. I have no idea what stimulated her to affirm her teen in this way, but I wish you could have seen her young man's face. He literally glowed. She had given him an incredible gift of affirmation.

It's amazing what just a sentence or a few words from us can mean in a teen's life. Remember how Hillary Clinton never forgot a dismissive comment from her father. Here are some cheers every parent can use:

- ❖ Have I told you recently how glad I am that you're my son [daughter]?
- ❖ Way to go!
- ❖ I can't believe how well you did on that test!
- ❖ Thanks for being nice to that girl in your youth group.
- ❖ I'm really glad you're trying out for the team.
- ❖ What a nice job you did cleaning up your room.
- ❖ Good job on your schoolwork. You're working hard.
- ❖ You're growing up to be so handsome!
- ❖ You're growing up to be so beautiful!
- ❖ God surely has someone special waiting for you.
- ❖ Look at those muscles! You are one strong boy!
- ❖ I'm impressed with your character.
- ❖ I prayed for you this morning, and I thanked God for you.
- ❖ We're so blessed God gave you to us to nurture.
- ❖ You're the most honest kid, really.
- ❖ Keep on doing a great job!

The bottom line is that you need to look for occasions when you can be your teen's best cheerleader. Become an expert at affirming and approving him or her. I can't stress enough how important your support is in helping your teens become highly healthy young adults who are prepared to go out into the world and become everything their Creator designed them to be.

BLAMELESS LOVE

Do you love your child blamelessly, unconditionally? Or is your love conditional, as in "I love you because of . . . " or "I love you if . . . "? Loving your teen because he gets good grades is conditional; loving your teen if she makes the swim team is provisional.

Here's a great test of unconditional love. Imagine what you'd say to your teen daughter if she and I had this conversation in my examination room:

Me: How can I help you today?
Her: Uh, I think I need a test.
Me: What kind of test?
Her: A pregnancy test.
Me: And why do you think you need this test?
Her (turning red): Because I've been having sex with my boyfriend, and
          I've missed a period.

I've delivered the life-changing news "the test results say you're pregnant" many times to unwed teens in my medical career. Fifty percent of the time one or both parents are in the room when I make this pronouncement. There have been times when I've felt all the oxygen sucked out of the room. The news almost always crushes the parents. In a few moments, their reactions run the gamut—from disbelief to anger to, finally, a grudging acceptance.

This is where the rubber meets the road. Will the parents love the child even at a moment like this? Is their love really unconditional? Or did their love change because their high school daughter got pregnant out of wedlock? I'm happy to report that most parents—I'd say around 80 percent—*do* love their daughter unconditionally during tough moments like this.

This is the time to draw close, not walk away. A time to hug, not abandon. A time to say, "I still love you," not "You stupid jerk! How could you do something like that?"

I know this is a worst-case scenario for any parent, but you have to mentally prepare yourself to love your teens unconditionally, to practice blameless, unconditional love early and often. Your foundation of parental love and support enables them to step out and grow to become the young men and women God created them to be. But your teens need informed, consistent, loving encouragement from you, not just empty praise. To provide this lifelong gift, you must know them well—be up to speed on who their friends are, who their teachers are, what classes they're taking, what's going on with their extracurricular activities, and what they're doing on weekend nights.

Love is the most basic of all emotional needs. God designed us to desire and seek out this kind of love. Thankfully, it's the type of love he extends to us. When you love teens in a healthy way, they feel as though they belong to something greater than themselves. They feel they have value and significance. Their feelings, thoughts, and opinions matter. Teens who know that God and their parents love them are more likely to become highly healthy.

Be careful, however. All love is not equal. Parents can choose between two kinds of love—*conditional love*, which is highly unhealthy, and *unconditional love*, which is highly healthy. Most parents—myself included—have used both kinds of love at one time or another, but the average parent leans toward expressing one. Wise parents are aware that they need to demonstrate unconditional love as often as they can.

Conditional (blaming) love requires a certain behavior or performance from teens in order to trigger the expression of love. They have to do something or be something in order to *earn* your love. One form of conditional love is "love if." If you're only expressing your love after your son catches a touchdown pass or your daughter gets a prime role in the school musical, they'll quickly pick up what pushes your "love if" button. Or there's the "love because" form of conditional love. If you only express your love if your son wears his hair a certain length or if your daughter is thin, they'll soon pick up that they are only worthy of your love because of something they are or are not. In essence, you blame them for not earning or deserving your love.

The alternative is unconditional love, which means you love your teen "in spite of"—even when he drops the game-winning pass in the end zone; you love your daughter even when she finds herself on the stage crew and not in the cast. It's putting an arm around a shoulder and saying, "Hey, you did your best. I'm so proud of the way you tried." Blameless love says to your teen, "There is nothing you can do to make me love you more. You will never lose my love."

Here are some things that say "unconditional love" to your teen:

❖   *Touch them.* You can touch your teen's heart through appropriate touch—a friendly pat on the shoulder, a toss of her hair, warm hugs, a nonsexual massage. Some parents think teens outgrow touch or can't bring themselves to make physical contact, but it's important to their emotional health. Touch says, "You are important to me and worthy of my interest and my time."

❖ *Find your teen's uniqueness.* Has your teen become good at something? Tennis? Basketball? Piano? Scottish dancing? Drama? Most likely, your teen has developed some sort of skill that sets him or her apart from peers.

❖ *If your teen doesn't have some special skill, don't sweat it.* It just means your teen hasn't yet discovered his or her special gift or talent, which is a gift from the Creator. Remember how delighted you were when you counted ten fingers and ten toes in the delivery room? Your child was normal. That's who he or she is. Love that special person like a special person, pointing out the pleasing character traits you see. As you do, you'll begin to see more and more clearly his or her incredible uniqueness.

CONNECTEDNESS

Author, physician, and Harvard psychiatrist Edward M. Hallowell believes that connection (what I call *connectedness*) is the most important part of the cycle children need in order to thrive. In other words, connectedness is foundational to our teens' becoming highly healthy. Connectedness to parents is the anchor; however, connectedness to friends, school activities, extracurricular activities, and even work (in the form of part-time jobs) makes up the mortar for building a highly healthy foundation for adulthood. This aspect of the ABCD's is so intertwined with relationships that I'll spend an entire chapter talking about it in part 4 (see page 231).

DISCIPLINE

We now come to the fourth letter—*D* for "Discipline." Lifting up our teens with affirmation, blameless love, and connectedness is critical for their health. But like a table, a fourth leg is needed to keep things on an equilibrium—the leg of parental guidance and enforced boundaries. If teens are to stay safe and healthy, your love must be balanced by and actively demonstrated through appropriate, loving discipline.

The term *discipline* has several meanings, and the nuances are worth examining. The dictionary's first definition of the noun *discipline* is "training that develops self-control, character, or orderliness and efficiency." Yet when most parents hear the word *discipline*, they equate it with "punishment," which is the fourth meaning given by the dictionary.

Just because your teens are nearing full physical maturation doesn't mean your days of parental discipline are over. Just the contrary. Teens still disobey, still act untrustworthy, and still display woeful attitudes around the house on occasion. Obviously, the old methods of discipline no longer work. You can't ask Johnny to stand in a corner or turn a rebellious teen over your knee for an old-fashioned spanking. Those days are long gone, but good discipline is absolutely necessary and helps teens learn to function in a highly healthy fashion.

Maintaining discipline will require occasional instances of punishment— and the more creative, the better. Telling your teen he can't see his friends ever again is over the top, but a Friday night without TV or videos or computer games will capture his attention. Extra chores around the house can send a message. And don't forget that teens who drive hate to lose the keys to the family car. Right discipline defines protective boundaries and reminds your teen that there will invariably be consequences for breaching those boundaries.

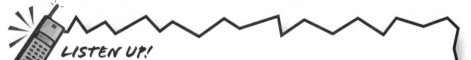

LISTEN UP!

Discipline your children while you still have the chance; indulging them destroys them.

Wise discipline imparts wisdom; spoiled adolescents embarrass their parents.

King Solomon in Proverbs 19:18; 29:15 (The Message)

Six Keys to Protecting Teens through Discipline

Long before I left my medical practice to work for Focus on the Family, I had read every Dr. Dobson book on how to raise children and be a good parent. Dr. Dobson articulated his classic principles so well I don't think you have to go anywhere else. Barb and I felt as though we were sitting at his feet whenever we read—and reread—a chapter from *Dare to Discipline* or *The Strong-*

Willed Child. From Dr. Dobson's writings, we found six key principles, which I outlined in *God's Design for the Highly Healthy Child* and apply here to teens:

1. Define the boundaries before they are enforced. Teens have the right to know what is and what is not acceptable behavior before they are held responsible for breaking the rules. You can't say "You have to be in by 11:00 p.m." and not tell your teens what the consequences are for being fifteen minutes late, thirty minutes late, or one hour late. If you're going to enforce curfew by the minute, then say so. If you're going to have a fifteen-minute grace period before they're officially late, then say so. Either way, let them know in advance what the consequences are for breaking curfew.

2. Avoid making impossible demands. Sure, all parents would love their kids to take AP courses, get high SAT scores, and have 4.0 report cards. But few teens are capable of being whizzes in the classroom. Even in this era of grade inflation, a straight-A report card is still a rare event in school these days. By the same token, some dads want to relive their glory days on the gridiron, so they place subtle pressure on their sons to be All-League football players when in actuality they contribute to the team in a backup role. Parents should set the bar, but it takes a thoughtful parent to place the bar just high enough to push his or her teen to greater heights without deflating the ego. Is your teen performing at a level that makes sense for his or her gifts and abilities? If so, you've set the bar at the right height.

3. Distinguish between irresponsibility and willful defiance. Teens can act goofy sometimes or like little Machiavellians. There's a difference between irresponsibility, such as leaving the car windows down overnight when a thunderstorm hits, and willful defiance, such as coming in after midnight when he knew full well he should have been home an hour earlier. This is an area where you can show grace—God's grace—as you effectively discern what your teen's motives were for his or her acts of negligence or defiance.

4. When defiantly challenged, respond with confident decisiveness. Intuitively you know the difference between irresponsibility and willful defiance, and when your teen has thrown down the gauntlet, you must respond in kind. Dr. Dobson suggests that when children "make it clear that they're looking for a fight, you would be wise not to disappoint them!" When nose-to-nose confrontations happen, it's extremely important to know ahead of time what you will do—and then to respond confidently.

5. Reassure and teach after the confrontation is over. Remember how you hugged your toddler after a spanking to let him know that everything was going to be all right? You don't spank teens, of course, but they still need to hear your reassurance that you love them. You may need to remind them of the ways they can avoid correction or punishment in the future. Teens never outgrow their need for reassurance after times of discipline.

6. *Let love be your guide!* It doesn't do any good to get into a shouting match. Sure, your teens will do things to make you angry, but you must keep your cool. During these few remaining years they live under your roof, you have a powerful opportunity to model adult ways of handling conflict, which will help them in the workplace and in their relationships in the future.

Parenting Style Makes a Huge Difference

I've closely followed the research of Diana Baumrind and other child development researchers who have studied the highly healthy characteristics of children. Here's a list of traits parents would love to see in their children:

- ❖ independence
- ❖ satisfaction
- ❖ maturity
- ❖ self-starting
- ❖ self-reliance
- ❖ self-control
- ❖ peace
- ❖ patience
- ❖ curiosity
- ❖ friendliness
- ❖ goodness
- ❖ kindness
- ❖ achievement orientation

The researchers attempted to identify the most significant elements of parenting style likely to foster these wonderful qualities. They found that a father's and a mother's parenting style captures two important elements: *parental responsiveness* and *parental demandingness*. Parental responsiveness (also referred to as parental warmth or supportiveness) refers to "the extent to which parents intentionally foster individuality, self-regulation, and self-assertion by being attuned, supportive, and acquiescent to children's special needs and demands." Parental demandingness (also referred to as behavioral control) refers to "the claims parents make on children to become integrated into the family whole, by their maturity demands, supervision, disciplinary efforts, and willingness to confront the child who disobeys."

I like to think that a balance of these two represents a balance of love and limits, which we must keep in mind as we move into a discussion of four dominant styles of parenting—each of which balances love and limits a bit differently. See the chart on page 179 for a summary of these styles.

Dictator Parents

These parents are domineering, autocratic, and highly controlling in their insistence that their children knuckle under to their authority. They rely on commands and value obedience as an absolute virtue. Dictator parents set iron-fisted limits and rules. Their teens do what they're told—or else. These parents are big on punishment (external force) instead of using discipline (coaching with both external force when necessary and helping the teens develop an internal sense of right and wrong). They either don't believe or can't be sure their teens will do the right thing when no one else is watching. Dictator parents do not encourage give-and-take with their teens. They never negotiate, and they take no prisoners. They demand that their children never express any disagreement with their decisions, decrees, or declarations.

Researchers have found that the children of dictator parents tend to lack social competence, have lower self-esteem, and rarely take the initiative in activities. They show less intellectual curiosity, are not spontaneous, and usually rely on the voice of authority.

When these teens leave home, they tend to drift either into the "top dog" or "bottom dog" category. They may become dictatorial bosses or submissive followers. They may become procrastinators—resistant to schedules and expectations—or they may push themselves and others unmercifully.

Champion Parents

Champion parents are warm and nurturing parents who administer blameless love. They communicate well with their children and balance love, grace, and mercy with clear authority. They dispense rewards and penalties appropriately. Champion parents stay cool, calm, collected, and in control. They expect mature behavior from their children, and when they see it, they affirm and even reward it. They see themselves as their children's guides and guardians, their providers and protectors, and their coaches and cheerleaders.

Champion parents are big on discipline as I define it—teaching and guiding rather than punishing and dominating their children. They respect their teens' independence and decisions as they grow older and mature. Nevertheless, these parents generally hold firm in their own positions. They are clear and explicit about their points of view but are equally willing to admit they are wrong or have made a mistake.

Best-Friend Parents

Best-friend parents are warm and accepting, just like champion parents, but they are extremely concerned about not stifling their child's creativity. Best-friend parents make few demands for mature behavior; they usually don't expect their wishes to be carried out. They are very much in tune with their children's emotional needs but have difficulty setting limits. Because of this, they tend to parent inconsistently and to resort to negotiating with their teens. Researchers call these parents indulgent and permissive, who, ironically, often become resentful of the teens they "loved" so much. They often end up feeling like martyrs.

Teens who have best-friend parents generally have difficulty controlling their impulses or accepting responsibility. They may be bored in the midst of the indulgence poured out on them. When these teens become young adults, they continue to expect others to give them what they want when they want it. These kids usually hate to work and as a result tend not to find or hold jobs. They have limited career goals and can fail to persist in life.

Marshmallow Parents

Marshmallow parents are uninvolved, and they demand little and respond minimally. These "whatever" parents are basically asleep at the wheel of parenting. Marshmallow parents raise teens who tend to be angry, rebellious, egocentric, selfish, and demanding—because they usually don't care either. These teens can have attachment, cognition, and emotional problems. They may lack in social skills and are more likely to be aggressive.

FYI . . .   ⏪ ▶ ⏸ ⏹ ⏩

▶ *A Parenting Style Case Study*

Imagine you're putting clothes into your teen's dresser. When you open the drawer, you see a pack of cigarettes. Here's how parents of the four parenting styles might react:

1. Dictator parents would erupt in a volcano of righteous indignation, saying something like, "Go throw these away this second!

Then come back in your room. You're grounded for a month. No phone. No friends can come over. You will not leave home except to go to school."

2. Champion parents would take a deep breath and perhaps recall one of their teen indiscretions. These parents would seize the opportunity to teach or coach their teen. They might say, "I know you want to grow up, and I know being independent and acting cool are important to you. But you know how unhealthy smoking is. You also know that the rule in our home is absolutely no smoking at anytime. Can we talk about it a bit?"

3. Best-friend parents would believe their teen should be allowed to express his or her impulses freely. Making this an issue could make things sticky, so they'd choose to pass by this opportunity to help their teen make a wise decision or solve a problem.

4. Marshmallow parents would overlook or ignore the incident—hoping against hope the problem would just go away.

When the teens nurtured in these parenting styles are evaluated, what do we see? As you might expect, champion parents come out on top. Their teens show the highest academic achievement, the highest social skills, and the fewest behavioral and psychosocial problems. These teens tend to be intellectually, emotionally, and relationally healthy.

Dictator parents and best-friend parents are in a tie for a very distant second place. Dictator parents have teens with the second-highest academic achievement, the second-lowest behavioral problems, the third-highest social skills, and the third-lowest psychosocial problems. Compare this to best-friend parents, who have teens with the second-highest social skills, the second-lowest psychosocial problems, the third-highest academic achievements, and the third-lowest behavioral problems.

Last and by far the least, marshmallow parents have teens with the lowest academic achievement, the lowest social skills, and the highest psychosocial and behavioral problems.

Go to page 179, where you can view a table that summarizes the four parenting styles.

Check It Out! ◄◄ ► ❙❙ ■ ►►

► Which parenting style do you lean toward? How about your spouse? If you'd like to determine your particular parenting style, you can find several self-tests on my website (www.highlyhealthy.net). If either or both of you aren't champions, you can seek resources to help you become a highly healthy parent (be sure to check out www.highlyhealthy.net). You can do your own quick assessment by looking back at the way you rated your teen's emotional wheel (pages 39–44). Add the points on the top and bottom vertical spokes. If the score is 6 or higher, you lean more toward the "parental responsiveness" category. Now add the points on the left- and right-hand horizontal spokes. If your score is 6 or higher, you lean more toward the "parental demandingness" category.

Looking at Scott's chart (page 52), Barb and I had 7 points in the vertical spokes of the emotional wheel (high in parental responsiveness) and 5 points in the horizontal spokes (borderline in parental demandingness). We would have made it into the "Champion Parents" category, but just barely. Yet we weren't satisfied. We knew we had work to do to increase the chances of Scott continuing as a highly healthy teen and becoming a highly healthy adult.

Balancing Love and Training

As your teens grow older, the need for discipline and the way discipline is administered change. If you're too soft—overemphasizing love and failing to teach obedience, your teens will disrespect you. If you're overly authoritarian and oppressive, your teens will shut you out of their lives. The goal is to balance love and training, mercy and fairness, warmth and firmness, tenderness and jurisdiction.

If you didn't mess up when you were a teen, you have nothing to worry about. Your teens will be perfect angels. Your days of maintaining discipline and training your teens are over. All you have to worry about is paying their college bills and saving money for their weddings. Then again, if you weren't perfect in high school—like yours truly—you can't expect your teens to sail through those years. I view any discipline during the teen years as midcourse corrections. Your teen is flying fast toward the target—adulthood—and you're handing him or her the plane's steering wheel for longer and longer stretches of time. You're still the captain, and there will be occasions when you need to take the controls during turbulent times.

You never know when it might happen. Our son, Scott, went off to college. He entered Samford University, located in Birmingham, Alabama, with nineteen units of college credit and a high grade point average. Since those nineteen units counted toward graduation, Scott assumed the high grades he earned with those credits would be dovetailed into his GPA at Samford. He's a bright young man, and he figured he could academically skate during his first semester. He didn't even make a 2.0, which means he had a few D's to go with his few C's.

THE FOUR PARENTING STYLES

	More Setting of Limits (demanding; high expectations; sets boundaries and limits)	Less Setting of Limits (undemanding; low expectations; sets no or few limits)
More Dispensing of Love (accepting and affirming; blameless love; responsive and cheerleaders)	**CHAMPION PARENTS** • authoritative • coach/cheerleader —connects • demanding but responsive • reasoned compliance	**BEST-FRIEND PARENTS** • responsive but undemanding • indulgent, permissive
Less Dispensing of Love (rejecting and unaffirming; conditional or blaming love; unresponsive or critical)	**DICTATOR PARENTS** • authoritarian • policeman/dictator —disconects • demanding but unresponsive • forced compliance	**MARSHMALLOW PARENTS** • unresponsive and undemanding • neglectful

The academic dean sent him a letter saying that if grades didn't improve the following semester, he wouldn't be allowed to register for classes again.

For some reason, Scott didn't think those academic standards applied to him. He had those A's and B's from those college courses he took in high school, right? Didn't those grades count? Nope. The dean was serious. When Scott continued to deliver grades south of the 2.0 border, Samford University declared him academically ineligible.

Scott's options were (1) dropping out and never coming back to Samford, (2) applying to another college and never coming back to Samford, or (3) taking a semester off and applying to be reinstated. If Scott chose the latter option, Samford wanted him to work or travel—to do something worthwhile. The reapplication process involved an interview and submitting an essay on what he had learned during his "sabbatical."

Scott wanted to come to Colorado Springs and live with us. Barb and I prayed about what we should do. I have to be honest: Barb wanted to allow him to come home, but I didn't think it'd be wise. We agreed he needed to understand there were consequences for his behavior. To be asked to sit out of college for a semester and land back in his cushy bedroom didn't sound like much of a consequence to us. So we practiced a little tough love. "Scott," I said, "you're going to have to find a place of your own and support yourself."

LISTEN UP!

Let me emphasize one point about physical punishment. I agree with the experts who teach that spanking should never (or only very rarely) occur after six to eight years of age. Teens deeply resent being hit or spanked. The former is child abuse; the latter makes them feel childish. Consequences must be creative, swift, and reasonable when compared to the offense. "You're grounded for the next six months!" is untenable when your teen arrives home a half hour late from bowling with friends. If you sprang for the evening, you might say, "The next time you'll have to pay for your bowling night."

Dr. Walt Larimore

He gulped. As he studied his options, Scott decided to move to our old hometown in Kissimmee, where he found a job as a substitute teacher at the high school he had attended. Then he found a place to live.

Here's one of the neat things that happened. A week or two after landing on his feet in Kissimmee, Scott gave Bill Judge a phone call. (If you recall, Bill was my mentor and accountability partner when we lived in Florida.)

"Mr. Judge, you know how you used to meet with my daddy every Tuesday morning and help him out?" Scott asked.

"Why yes, I sure do," Bill replied.

"Would you meet with me every Tuesday morning?"

I thought that was so cool when I heard about it. Scott had seen mentoring lived out by me, and now he decided he wanted the same type of accountability during a pivotal moment in his life.

Scott served his sentence, so to speak, and returned to Samford a changed young man. That's called staying the course—for him and for us.

What Scott went through was a mild form of rebellion. He wanted to do what he wanted to do. He experienced the consequences of his actions, and I'm sure he'll never forget the lesson. Some teens, however, aren't interested in mild rebellion. They're interested in partying and getting high. Taking drugs is a huge lure for teens, and in the next chapter I'll examine the reasons and suggest some actions to take if you suspect your teen is caught up in the drug scene.

Chapter 9

ESCAPE INTO ECSTASY

Our family lived in the Orlando area during the 1990s, the decade that solidified its reputation as the party crossroads of the world. Every day, thousands of teens and young adults disembarked from wide-bodies landing at Orlando International—flying in from every state in the Union and around the world. They were in a party mood from the minute they hit the Jetway, primed to enjoy Central Florida's year-round warm weather and its proximity to Walt Disney World, Epcot Center, Universal Studios, Sea World, and other resorts.

Partying after-hours in their Days Inn room wasn't fun; they wanted to paint the town red. To meet the demand, nightclubs such as the Firestone Club, Metropolis, and Matrix sprang up like spring mushrooms, offering a blend of pulsating, frenetic music and alluring lighting to foster an atmosphere of—how else should I put it?—hedonism. The beefy bouncers holding the red rope at the front door were ostensibly bound to bar underage minors from entering. Sometimes the flimsy fake IDs merited entrance, but other times a bouncer's head jerk told them to move on.

With so many teens looking to party hearty, enterprising promoters sniffed a business opportunity. Why not give them somewhere to go? Better yet, a place where there were no rules and no restrictions. A place where they could get stoned out of their minds and no one would care.

Adopting a trend that started in the English countryside outside London and Manchester during the late 1980s, these promoters began staging "raves" in the greater Orlando area. They would rent a rusty-roofed warehouse in the industrial district for an evening, wire it up with state-of-the-art computerized lighting, truck in a monster sound system, hire a DJ, set up booths to sell

booze, and employ some down-and-outers as security. After papering the local
high schools, record stores, coffee shops, and malls with fliers advertising their
"Pandemonium" rave, the promoters would sit back and collect ten or twenty
bucks from every hopped-up teen pushing to gain entrance. What a money-
maker! Orlando raves drew *thousands* in a single night, many drawn by its all-
inclusive philosophy of PLUR—Peace, Love, Unity, and Respect.

I've never witnessed a rave, but from what I hear, it's like entering Dante's
Inferno. It's pitch-dark inside, except in the middle of the dance floor, where
colorful lights and computerized lasers move with the techno music cranked
up to jet aircraft–decibel levels. On the dance floor, a sweaty soup of kids
gyrates every which way. Many ravers perform "freaking" dances that simu-
late sexual intercourse—grinding each other as they dip up and down in syn-
chronization. Others pretend they have a beach ball between them, which they
suggestively and seductively form with their hands. That practice is called "liquid dancing," and it's indicative of the anything-goes atmosphere that permeates raves. You won't find bow-tied chaperones touching shoulders and
telling young couples to break it up at these dances.

Raves advertise a 10:00 p.m. or 11:00 p.m. start time, but no respectable
raver would ever show up before midnight. Given the late hour, many teens
arrive BOA—blitzed on arrival. They rave all night until dawn, which gives
them plenty of time to take more drugs and buy more drinks. It's a dealer's
selling field inside the rave. He's retailing hits of heroin, Rohypnol ("roofies"),
GHB, crystal meth, and ecstasy, often at a 3,000 percent markup. Synthetic
drugs like GHB and ecstasy are made locally, which means they don't have the
overhead costs associated with drugs smuggled into the country, such as pot
and heroin. At $20 to $40 a pill for something that cost pennies to make, he's
raking it in.

Ecstasy is the most popular of the recent designer drugs to sweep through
the teen culture. Scientists call it methylene-dioxymethamphetamine, or
MDMA, but on the street it became known as "ecstasy." Producers like to
imprint ecstasy pills with Nike swooshes or color them in Crayola colors. The
pills, which are about the size of an aspirin, can be ingested orally, but the
drug's "benefits" don't kick in for a half hour or so. Studies indicate that even
the first dose of ecstasy can begin destroying the brain cells crucial to memory and sleep. Each additional hit does more and more potentially permanent damage.

If you haven't heard of ecstasy, don't feel bad. Many parents haven't. It's a
semisynthetic compound, first patented by a German drug company in 1913

as an appetite suppressant. While the use of cocaine and marijuana has stabilized in many countries, the use of ecstasy is increasing exponentially. For example, U.S. Customs seized more than 9 million doses in 2002, compared to less than 400,000 in 1997. The international network that smuggles the drug is huge and well organized because of the high demand.

And it's in high demand because ecstasy users get quite a high. They're hit with a burst of energy and an overwhelming desire to touch or hug others. Called the "hug drug," teens intensify the high when they receive body massages or engage in sexual activity. Kids spiked on ecstasy are said to be "rolling" or "peaking" because it raises the heart rate, blood pressure, and body temperature. Since ecstasy is chemically related to amphetamines—chemical uppers—their entire metabolism kicks into high gear. Kids don't feel hungry or tired, which explains why they can dance and act crazy until the sun comes up. But they dehydrate quickly, and quite often users will, without knowing it, grind their teeth or bite their tongues. Those who have a bad reaction to ecstasy have been known to drop to the ground and flop like a fish out of water, vomiting and spitting up foam.

JAKE'S STORY

My first encounter with ecstasy was with a male patient who struck me as your average Christian high school sophomore. Jake didn't have a clue where he'd go to college, nor did any thoughts rumble through his head about what he wanted to do with his life. He had joked to his mom, "I feel the Lord is calling me to be a billionaire!"

Jake loved his summer job as a lifeguard at a nearby community pool and was active in sports, student organizations at school, and his church group. He said he first took the "hug drug" at a friend's house after church one night. He was curious about ecstasy because he had heard friends talking about it at school—including his Christian buddies. They said ecstasy made them feel closer to God and to each other.

The first time he popped a "Smurf pill," nothing happened for the first fifteen minutes or so, but then the effects kicked in. He began to feel happy. He felt an incredible love for the other guys in his group, and the sleeves of his shirt felt plush and soft. That night, his pal Randy—who'd also taken a hit of ecstasy—came over and wrapped him in a bear hug. He'd never done anything like that before. Jake said Randy was normally the biggest worrywart in the world, but that night he was all touchy-feely, although in a good way. They talked and shared as never before. They even had an awesome prayer time, Jake said.

The first high was so great he couldn't wait to take it again. "I felt so ener-gized and so restored in my relationship with God!" he said, adding that what he liked about the drug was that there were no side effects and he couldn't get hooked to it. "Doc, I know I'm not addicted," he said. "I can stop anytime. It's just that ecstasy has helped me to know God and to like myself."

Jake told me all this from his hospital bed inside a psychiatric hospital, where I was doing a medical consultation for his psychiatrist. He landed there after taking ecstasy at an all-night rave party. The drug caused Jake to ignore the body's warning signals that he needed rest and water. He literally danced himself into a heatstroke and collapsed. After paramedics rushed him to the hospital, his parents and youth pastor received the shocks of their lives when they learned he had been taking ecstasy. He confessed that he had been using ecstasy several times a week—a reminder that "church kids" aren't immune to the siren call of drugs.

I'm happy to report that medical intervention and intensive treatment turned Jake around, and he remained drug-free after he checked out of the psychiatric hospital. I had the privilege of being his physician during high school and into college. I saw him grow spiritually in many ways without the "help" of ecstasy. He learned from this experience, and thankfully he's shown no evidence of brain damage. During college, he volunteered at a ministry that helped other kids and their parents who were struggling with drug abuse.

Though Jake was nurtured in a Christian home, it didn't shield him from the danger of drugs. Yet, statistically speaking, teens nurtured in Christian homes and involved in church activities are *less* likely to become involved with drugs. Young people who consider religion to be an important part of their lives are half as likely to try marijuana, for instance, or any dangerous substances that can lead to addiction. In a 1999 Gallup Poll, more than half of teens said that religion helps them deal with problems related to drugs and alcohol.

In many ways, church youth programs—Wednesday night activities, retreats, missions outreach projects, and summer camps—are effective forms of substance abuse prevention. In fact, after the influence of parents, a teen's relationship with God and with a faith community is one of the most power-ful anti-drugs. It all has to do with the connectedness I talked about in the previous chapter. Young people are encouraged to avoid doing drugs from voices other than your own, and they're being instilled with moral and spiri-tual values that will help them resist drugs.

> FYI...

> ▶ Drug abuse can affect the body's neurotransmitters. Brain chemicals such as serotonin can lead to mood disturbances when they're out of balance. Even single doses of ecstasy can impact the serotonin level in the brain, which means it's possible that kids could be thrown into a fairly dramatic depression after just one evening with ecstasy.

JUST A LITTLE SQUEEZE

Jake was one of the fortunate ones—and he's lucky he's not a girl. Teen girls are more at risk when they take party drugs like ecstasy and GHB because it makes them vulnerable to being sexually abused, often by someone they've never met. The date rape drug of choice these days is GHB, which stands for gamma-hydroxybutyrate. Detective Scott Perkins, who used to be an undercover cop with the Orlando Police Department, said that sexual predators will fill a Visine bottle with GHB and go into a rave, looking for attractive girls. They see one they like, strike up a conversation, and when she isn't looking, squirt some GHB into her drink.

GHB works in three stages. In the first stage, she feels sexually aggressive and comes on to a guy. The second stage is when she says she doesn't feel so good. The third stage is when she passes out. The guy who doses her knows all the stages. As soon as she complains about not feeling good, he suggests taking her outside for some "fresh air." By the time they get outside the rave, he's got her. She's done for.

I've read hundreds of victim statements over the years. The typical statement is a young woman or teen girl stating that she was hanging out at a rave or a nightclub, and then she met a guy with black hair named Johnny who asked her to dance. After the dance, he offered to buy her a drink, and the next thing she knew, she woke up under the fire escape with her pants off and a pain in her thighs.

But teens don't need to leave home to get high. Diane Stem of Nashville, Tennessee, was among the unaware until her sixteen-year-old son, Ricky, died suddenly on June 20, 1996, after huffing Freon from the air conditioner in his room. "We had never heard of huffing before Ricky died. We never thought to warn him," she said. "Ricky invited a killer into his room. He didn't know. It was supposed to be harmless fun."

Substance abuse experts report we're at the beginning of what they consider to be a silent epidemic: the use by children of common household products as inhalants. It is a public health problem that remains off the radar of most parents and doctors.

According to the Office of National Drug Control Policy (ONDCP), one teen in five has tried sniffing fumes of legal household goods by the end of high school. Kids call this "huffing"—inhaling the vapors from household products ranging from nail polish remover to aerosol whipped cream. It affects 12 million American teens. Edward Jurith, acting director of the ONDCP, notes, "These items can be deadly, but they are right under our kids' noses everyday. When kids sniff or huff, they are inhaling poisons that do real damage, or even kill them."

In 1998, nearly a million teens tried huffing for the first time. Inhalants are the most popular recreational drug among twelve-year-olds, according to the Substance Abuse and Mental Health Services Administration's most recent National Household Survey. In addition, almost half a million young people use inhalants in any given month. According to the survey, there were an estimated 991,000 new inhalant users in 1998, up from 390,000 in 1990. And the number is still growing. A 2002 survey reported an estimated 1,125,000 new inhalant users in 2001.

You may think your home is not at risk. But it may well be, given the fact that products that can be toxic when sniffed include room deodorizers, correction fluid, shoe polish, nitrous oxide, paint thinner, spray paints, and other aerosol sprays. In fact, more than a thousand different household substances can be inhaled to provide a brief high, according to the National Inhalant Prevention Coalition.

Symptoms of inhalant abuse, besides failing grades, chronic school absences, and general apathy, can include paint or stains on body or clothing; chemical-soaked rags, bags, or socks; spots or sores around mouth; red or runny eyes or nose; chemical breath odor; and intoxicated appearance. Long-term effects can include short-term memory loss, hearing loss, limp spasms, permanent brain damage, bone marrow damage, liver and kidney damage, and death—just to name a few. And, worst of all, death can occur even with the first use. While there is no way to tell which child will succumb or how many sniffing sessions it will take, statistics indicate that those who do not suffer illness may go on to try other drugs. (More information is available at www.inhalants.org.)

DRUG-PROOFING YOUR TEENS

Now that I've scared you half to death, how can we equip our kids to resist peer pressure to use drugs?

Let Your Teen Know That You Know about Drugs

The time to start talking to your teens about drugs is the same time you should be talking about sex—way before puberty. If you haven't yet done so, you can still play catch-up by establishing a clear family position on drug use. You can play off the teachable moments that crop up during the day—the news on the radio that a Hollywood star died of a drug overdose or a famous celebrity checked into a drug treatment facility. Remind your teens that using drugs can destroy their health *now*—not at some nebulous time in the future. If they've been good students and have been talking about college, point out that admission counselors cast a wary eye toward applicants with a history of drug busts on their record.

Reading this book is one way you can get prepared to know the facts about certain drugs like ecstasy and GHB. If one of your children asks a question you can't answer, admit you don't know but resolve to find the answer. You'll find many answers to questions about drugs on my website (go to www .highlyhealthy.net).

This is not the time to talk down to your teens. Remember, they're probably feeling some degree of peer pressure to experiment, and teens will do almost anything to be accepted by their group. Let them know it's still cool to say no, to let that joint pass by, but then they should be looking for new friends. The old lament "your friends can bring you down" still applies today. I recall Barb quoting a proverb to our children when they were younger: "Don't respond to the stupidity of a fool; you'll only look foolish yourself."

Barb and I wanted our children to understand from an early age that the decisions they made would affect not only the rest of their own lives but also the lives of their children and their children's children. The decision to take drugs certainly was part of that equation. We talked constantly about what the experts call "risky behavior" but what the Bible calls "foolish decisions."

King Solomon of Israel once wrote, "Death is the reward of an undisciplined life; your foolish decisions trap you in a dead end."

We made our expectations very clear: "You do not try any drug at any time for any reason. You refuse the first time and every time. If you find yourself in an uncomfortable situation, call me or Mom immediately, and we'll come to get you—whenever and wherever." We also wanted our kids to know there would be consequences to using drugs—not only long term but in the short term as well. It was "one strike and you're out!" We took to heart what Solomon wrote: "Young people are prone to foolishness and fads; the cure comes through tough-minded discipline."

Tell Your Teen How Stupid You Were to Experiment with Drugs

If you, like Barb and me, didn't smoke marijuana or use street drugs growing up, I salute you, but we are in a minority. Many of today's parents of teens came of age in the 1970s, when drugs in high school were as common as bell-bottoms and Birkenstocks. You may have experimented to find out what all the hullabaloo was about. If you did, you may feel you'd be a hypocrite if you were to warn your teens about drugs. Take heart from this public service ad from the Partnership for a Drug-Free America:

> So you smoked pot. And now your kid's trying it and you feel like you can't say anything. Get over it. Pot can affect the brain and lead to more serious drug use. So you have to set the rules and expect your kid to live drug free, no matter how hypocritical it makes you feel. Because to help them with their problem, first you have to get over yours. To find out more, call 800-788-2800 or visit theantidrug.com.

Pretty cool, eh? So talk to your teen from your heart about what you did. Don't glorify your actions ("I got stoned so often I could have starred in *Fast Times at Ridgemont High*") or boast that the drugs didn't have any effect. They did, and you have to live with it the rest of your life. Tell your teen you want to spare him or her the pain you experienced. Drugs (and alcohol) alter your mind, which is why the Bible says not to drink in such a way as to change your thinking or behavior.

If someone in your family had a problem with drugs, don't try to hide it from your teen. Perhaps this family member can share how doing drugs messed up his or her life for a long time. Experience is a strong teacher, which is why parental influence is so important.

My brother Rick is a recovering alcoholic. I'm proud not only that he's been sober for seventeen years but that he helps others deal with their alcoholism. When Scott was younger, I asked Rick to share his story with my son. That evening was a real eye-opener. Scott heard firsthand the pain and consequences of addicting behavior. He and Rick have been very close since that evening, and I'm convinced my brother's story has helped my son say no when he was asked to take a drink or take a hit.

Don't Think That Taking Your Teen to the Doctor for a Drug Test Will Fix the Problem

You would think I'd be a big fan of drug tests, but I'm not. By the time most teens see me, the drugs have passed through their system. So a negative test doesn't tell you much.

When a mom dragged her son into the examination room and announced, "We need a drug test, Doctor," my antennae would usually shoot up. That child had become what we medical people call an "identified patient." The family identified the teen as a problem child, a black sheep who was using drugs, running away from home, or one detention away from getting kicked out of school. They had identified him as a bad kid.

I believe a small amount of teen drug use is experimentation, but more often than not, taking drugs is a cry for help. Something is amiss in the family, and doctors will not solve it in a five-minute office visit or by taking a urine sample. My tack was to refer them to a Christian psychologist or pastor for counseling, where the counselor could deal with the deep family issues that almost always underlie these situations.

The only time I'd do a "you shouldn't do drugs, Johnny" lecture was in cases where I felt what happened was a single case of experimentation. For instance, Johnny was talked into going to a rave in downtown Orlando, and he took a little pill. He came home at 5:00 a.m. zonked out. Five hours later, he was in my office, and bingo—I'd tell Johnny he had gone down the wrong road the night before, but let's hope it was a detour. I'd also, with his permission, hook him up with other teens in a local church youth group who would be able to minister to him and connect in a way I could not.

Let me also say I'm not a fan of home drug tests, except in those isolated instances where a teen is coming out of rehab or counseling, and he or she wants some kind of accountability. Home drug tests or random drug tests out of my office can act as a motivator to stay clean. In most cases, however, home drug tests cause parents and teen to pit themselves against each other instead of working together to get at the root of the problem.

LISTEN UP!

Teens can smell a hypocrite like they can smell a fast-food restaurant a block away. Are you medicating yourself with mood-altering pills, supplements, or alcohol? Are you using someone else's medications, or are you abusing medications (even if you get them on a doctor's prescription)? Do you come home from work and announce to the world that you need a drink to start the evening off right?

Dr. Walt Larimore

DON'T MISS THOSE SIGNPOSTS!

It's mind-boggling how many parents have sat in my office and said, "If only I had known!" It's easy to understand that lament. We brought these creatures into the world and watched them grow up; it's painful to picture them smoking joints and popping pills and acting crazy with their friends—but that's just what some of them do.

Hindsight is always 20/20, and many of these parents, upon reflection, admit they could have done a better job of picking up signs that their sons or daughters were getting into drugs.

It's pretty obvious that it takes money to acquire drugs. Drug dealers are probably the least altruistic creatures on earth, and they rarely extend credit, especially to flaky teens. Where is the money coming from? If your teen receives an allowance, is he or she asking for cash advances? Have you noticed occasions when you had less cash in your wallet than you thought you had? If your teen has a part-time job, does he or she ever put any money in the bank? Here's an interesting statistic: stressed-out, bored teens who receive $25 or more in pocket money each week are three times more likely to smoke, get drunk, and use drugs than peers without this cocktail of risk factors, according to a survey by the National Center on Addiction and Substance Abuse.

Other signs flash brighter than a Vegas hotel on the Strip. A sudden drop in GPA during the last semester. Lots of phone calls after 10:00 p.m. Sleeping in on Saturday until afternoon or being practically comatose when you try to wake them up for Sunday morning church. Dressing a *lot* different from the way they dressed a few months ago. Any sort of drug paraphernalia in their bedrooms. (Rolling papers, roach clips, and bongs are so seventies. Look for M&M or Skittles bags, which contain ecstasy pills, not melt-in-your-mouth chocolate. Baby pacifiers are popular with ecstasy users to protect them from grinding their teeth or biting their tongues.)

Does your teen seem to be spending the night regularly at a friend's house? That's often a tip-off. Even if the other parents are trustworthy, your teen and his friend could be sneaking out after midnight to hit the local rave or to meet up with some buddies to do drugs.

If you see these and other warning signs, plan on talking to your child when you're feeling calm and not rushed. Avoid direct accusations and "how dare you do this to me!" or "how could you disappoint me?" statements. Flying off the handle will drive your teen away. Plus, if you discover later that your teen was *not* using drugs, you'll find yourself with a damaged relationship that will be challenging to repair.

FYI . . .

▶ I've often had parents ask me, "Should I search my child's room?" I replied that Barb and I wanted our children to know that we *always* reserved the right to search their rooms at any time and for any reason. Period.

That said, we also understood the need for our teens to trust us, to depend on us to love and protect them, and to give them privacy in their room, so it was a balancing act for us. We believed it was important to respect a child's right to privacy—but only up to a point. If we had harbored any suspicions about drug use or another harmful activity, we would have first talked to our teen about it, seeking reassurance that there was no funny business going on. If we had ever judged that the situation had reached a point where we had to search our child's room, we would have had our child present during the search.

Think about what may be happening psychologically when a teen "accidentally" leaves something out on a desk, giving a parent an "invitation" to look. A teen wrestling with a problem will often leave clues behind—usually subconsciously. It's a way of communicating a need for help, because if a teen really wants to hide something, he or she can almost always do so successfully.

What if your teen won't talk to you about your concerns? Calmly let him or her know you're concerned about what's going on in his or her life and you'll be talking to other people, such as teachers, coaches, friends, and the school's guidance counselor. When you talk to others, you don't have to focus on your concerns about drugs. Just ask whether they've noticed anything unusual about your teen. If you hear anything that deepens your suspicions, bring the information to your teen.

Be sure to enforce discipline for any violation of agreed-on house rules. My rule of thumb is that parents should give their teens more freedoms, rights, and privileges as they demonstrate they can handle them. If school grades slip, however, parents shouldn't hesitate to reinstate rules, restrictions, and consequences that they've eased up on.

The same sort of structured rule system should be applied to a child who is using drugs. A teen who drinks should, for example, lose car privileges. If your teen doesn't uphold his or her end of an agreement, back up a little on the freedom you've given. Regaining your trust is then up to your teen. When you believe that your child is no longer using drugs and can be trusted again, you can ease up on the restrictions. You may want to consider enforcing a curfew (if you haven't done this before) or switching him or her to a new school (according to a 2003 study, children at Christian and secular private schools are far likelier to be drug free than those at public schools).

If you're running into a brick wall and your teen refuses to respond to you, seek help promptly. Meet with your pastor or family doctor and describe what you've seen. They will undoubtedly have names of people to contact. Ask for referrals to professionals and organizations with which the pastor or doctor has had direct experience.

If you think your teen is lying, and the evidence of drug use is strong, have your child evaluated by a professional counselor experienced with substance abuse. Be sure to stress to your teen that this isn't a punishment. Emphasize that you love your child, want to protect him or her, and desire the best help available. If you learn that your child's problem is serious enough to warrant admission to a drug treatment program, then swallow hard and do it. A good program will help the teen, the family, and you. As your son or daugh-ter works with skilled counselors, you'll be able to find support and comfort among other parents who walk a similar path.

Finally, I believe one of the major reasons teens turn to drugs is that they have a spiritual hole in their hearts. If teens can find a greater purpose for liv-ing, a reason larger than themselves not to take drugs, they tend to avoid abus-ing drugs. I'm convinced that Jesus Christ is the only one who can fill that hole in their hearts. Teens need a personal relationship with Christ more than ever when they're trying to get off drugs. Pray they'll be drawn by Christ's love. Pray that the Lord will bring godly people into their lives. Pray that their lives will be turned around.

HOME MEDICATIONS

Let's deal now with a different type of drug use among teens—prescrip-tion drugs taken for a variety of mental health ailments that include depres-sion, bipolar disorder, and attention deficit/hyperactivity disorder (ADHD).

I have no doubt we're in the middle of a mental health epidemic with teens. Nearly 30 percent of high school students said they felt sad almost every day for two consecutive weeks, according to a Youth Risk Survey. Bipolar dis-order, characterized by episodes of depression and mania that cause extreme shifts in mood and energy, affects 2.3 million adults in this country. Experts say that ADHD affects 3 percent to 5 percent of school-age children and two to three times as many boys as girls.

More on ADHD

Why are we hearing about so many cases of ADHD these days? To be sure, the diagnostic criteria are more refined than previously, which means we're diagnosing kids with ADHD we were overlooking ten to twenty years ago. But we're also seeing more misdiagnoses of ADHD, especially in white, middle-class boys who exhibit a variety of hyperactive, acting-out symptoms. In these cases, they are not truly ADHD kids, but they're often put on med-ications such as Ritalin or Adderall anyway. So we have a combination of bet-ter diagnoses and a preponderance of overdiagnoses of ADHD.

I recommend to parents that if you've either had a diagnosis of ADHD for your child or you think your child may have this disorder, be sure to seek a sec-ond opinion, especially from a child behavior team that is familiar with

ADHD. It may mean traveling to another town, or seeing a child psychiatrist or a primary care physician who specializes in child behavior, or visiting the mental health team at the children's hospital in your city. It's important to follow up, because roughly half of children who are appropriately diagnosed with ADHD have a "co-morbid" condition, which means there's something else going along with it—possibly a learning disorder or a depressive disorder.

One thing that surprises parents when I talk about this topic is that teens who are not diagnosed and properly treated for ADHD have outcomes that are worse in many areas than outcomes for those who are treated. Untreated teens are often out of the house seeking stimuli, and they tend to engage in more risky behavior. They are more likely to abuse drugs, smoke cigarettes, drink alcohol, and engage in sexual activity than kids who are treated. They are poor performers in school, get into more car accidents, and are prone to become more involved in criminal activity.

LISTEN UP!

The behavioral treatments for my patients with ADHD (and with any mental health issue) always involved the whole family. I wanted every family member to understand ADHD because it affects both siblings and parents, and it requires different parenting skills. Gaining this understanding is important, because teachers often view kids with ADHD as problem kids. Classmates see them as different and may mock their inability to sit still. Teens have a way of fulfilling expectations. If they are viewed by you as some sort of problem, they might give up in the classroom, academically and socially.

Dr. Walt Larimore

Carla's Story

Most teens don't outgrow ADHD. The good news is that ADHD is highly treatable these days, thanks to the dramatically positive effects of medications such as Ritalin, Dexedrine, Adderall, Concerta, Straterra, Wellbutrin, and others. I've seen teens' lives take dramatic turns once they got on meds. Their school performance often skyrockets, and their self-image takes off.

I remember treating a teen named Carla, an incredibly gifted person. She was the class clown—the student who couldn't stay in her seat, always looked out the window, never stayed on task, and couldn't focus on her schoolwork. When her grades slipped to C's and D's, her mom became concerned and brought her in to see me.

I ordered a battery of tests and learned that she was a classic hyperactive ADHD kid. I used a combination of behavioral therapy and medication therapy, trying two or three different medications before sensing that the third one was a home run. Carla's ability to focus in the classroom and on her schoolwork soared. Her grades shot up, and she nailed her SAT, coming in around 1300. Pretty good for a girl struggling to make D's at one time.

On a subsequent visit, Carla made an interesting statement: "Dr. Walt, my friends have asked me not to take my medication because they say I was more fun before."

"That's interesting," I said. "Let's talk about that. You have your old self and your new self. Which one do you prefer?"

Carla thought for a moment. "It would have to be my new self," she said. "I'm happier at school and doing better, but I do miss being called the class clown."

We shared a laugh, and I wished her the best. To this day, I'm glad her mom and dad loved her enough to have her evaluated.

Check It Out!

▶ For more on ADHD and various treatment options, check out *Why A.D.H.D. Doesn't Mean Disaster*. You can also learn more at my website (www.highlyhealthy.net).

More on Emotional Disorders

In many cases where a teen struggles with emotional turmoil, the parents are doing things right—helping their teen stay physically healthy, eat properly, get enough rest, develop a spiritual foundation, cultivate healthy relationships with others, and the like—and yet the emotional wheel still becomes unbalanced. Sometimes anxiety and depression disorders have genetic roots—they run in the family. I remember examining a young teen gymnast. Angie was an elite athlete who made the U.S. national team before her performances in the gym and in the classroom started dropping off. She had difficulty sleeping, difficulty with her appetite, and difficulty staying motivated to work hard. Her parents noticed the tailspin, so they brought her in to see me.

I went through my checklist. Her relationship wheel with her parents and friends looked great. Her physical wheel looked fine: she tested negative for anemia, iron deficiency, and thyroid condition, among other things. She had a deep spiritual foundation. But when I gave her a test for depression, the results were way off the scale. She clearly was in severe clinical depression.

I did some background checking. It turned out that her mother, grandmother, and aunt had all been treated (or were still being treated) for depression. All of them had manifested depression in their teen years. So Angie's situation was a case of a genetic depression syndrome called dysthymia, a low-grade depression that can be inherited.

I prescribed a mild antidepressant, and two weeks later, she was a different kid. Her mood had improved, her depression score was nearly normal, and her motivation had shot back up. In other words, she made a dramatic recovery.

Parents, if you're seeing evidence of a flattened emotional wheel in your teen and you suspect something isn't right, make an appointment right now with your family doctor or with a mental health counselor to have your son or daughter checked for depression or ADHD.

The Power of the Prescription Pad

I'd be remiss as a Christian doctor if I didn't tell you about another way to fight some depression cases. I learned it from psychiatrist Paul Meier, founder of the Meier Clinics, who told me one time that he often suggested to his patients that they memorize Scripture. I must admit I was surprised to hear this, and I asked if he did that just for his Christian patients. "No," he replied. "It works for my non-Christian patients too. The Word of God is powerful."

What Paul said that day got me thinking. A few days later, I was back in the office seeing patients. One was Debbie, a woman in her thirties I'd seen several times. She had the blahs, she said—no energy, no willingness to keep pressing on.

I figured she was depressed. It was in her family history. Her mother was depressed; her grandmother was depressed. I concluded that she—like the elite swimmer Angie—suffered from dysthymia, a low-level depression.

I talked with Debbie about various ways to treat her depression, and then I remembered what Paul Meier had told me. After describing the plan, I asked whether she'd be willing to try it.

"It sounds interesting to me," she said.

"Me too!" I agreed.

Then I had another idea. I reached for my prescription pad, and I wrote legibly (please, no jokes about doctor's handwriting!) the words "Memorize Psalm 1." I signed my name, and I wrote a second prescription for a prescription antidepressant.

"I'll see how you're doing in ten to fourteen days," I said.

At her next visit, I walked in, only to be greeted by a happy patient who insisted on hugging me.

"My, we must be feeling better," I remarked.

"I sure do, Doctor," Debbie replied with a bright smile.

"Let's have you complete this little test," I said, referring to a screening for depression. When I went through her score, the results were normal. (In my medical experience, this wasn't rare, but it was unusual.) *This is interesting*, I thought. *Is this really true, or is she faking her answers?*

"You seem like a different woman."

"You know, I really am. That prescription you gave me really worked."

"Yup, it really does. The antidepressant usually takes three or four days before it kicks in, sometimes three or four weeks, but I'm glad it's working for you."

"What are you talking about?"

"The medicine I prescribed for you."

"Doctor, I didn't fill that prescription. I filled the other one. I started reading my Bible every day, and I memorized Psalm 1."

"You did?"

"Yeah." And then she quoted Psalm 1.

"You really think it made a difference?" I asked.

"Just getting into God's Word and being able to meditate on it during the day blew me away," she said.

It blew me away too. I know that writing "Memorize Psalm 1" on a prescription pad will never be embraced by the medical community as a cure for depression. It just happened to be effective in Debbie's case. There are many treatment options—research has shown, for example, that exercise and exposure to natural sunlight can help lessen depression. The point I want to make is that medication, while effective, isn't the only option used for treating all cases of depression.

Check It Out!   ◀◀ ▶ ❚❚ ■ ▶▶

▶ For a medically reliable and biblically sound guide to understanding depression, finding help for it, experiencing hope in the midst of it, and discovering gifts and insights as a result of the struggle, I recommend *New Light on Depression*, written by David B. Biebel and Harold G. Koenig. Learn more about this book at my website (www.highlyhealthy.net).

LIGHTING UP

Although we were known as a faith-based practice in Kissimmee, Florida, we strove to be nonjudgmental with our patients. The philosophy and theology behind it was that Jesus sent the Holy Spirit to be the convictor, but he didn't send the church to convict people. We wanted to love people wherever they were in their life's journey.

For instance, whenever I was taking a patient's regular history, I always asked, "Do you use any tobacco products at all, or have you in the last year?"

That's a direct question, especially for a ninth-grader. If he or she would say no, I'd reply, "That's great, because one of the most dangerous things you can do is use tobacco products. There's nothing healthy about it. At your age, you're more likely to get addicted compared to someone who is older, so I'm proud of you for choosing not to do it."

Sometimes when I asked teens if they used tobacco products in the last year, I heard a distinct "Umm"—and that almost always meant a yes—or some shrugged their shoulders and nodded. In that case, I said, "You know it's dangerous, right?"

"Yup. I know it's dangerous."

"You've seen the pictures of the black lungs and people dying, right?"

"Yup."

"Are you ready to stop?"

"No, probably not."

"Well, if you ever want to stop, let me know. I can help you."

Then I'd ask about it at the next visit, and the next and the next. I wanted them to know I was there and ready to help whenever they were ready, whenever they really wanted to quit.

Surveys of teen smoking are sending smoke signals of distressing news. A White House–sponsored survey of cigarette smoking among sixth- through twelfth-graders found that cigarette use increased slightly to 27 percent in the 2002–2003 school year, up from 26 percent from the year before. Survey results were based on a sample of 110,000 students in twenty-four states.

It bothers me that smoking is popular in Hollywood. I'd like to be invited to a film studio boardroom so I could ask Hollywood executives why they push smoking in movies. Have we forgotten that smoking causes lung cancer and emphysema and will prematurely kill at least one-third of those who take up the despicable habit? Apparently so in Tinseltown.

Scientists from the Dartmouth Medical School said that teens' watching their favorite stars smoking in movies was an important factor in getting them to begin smoking. The study also said that the incidence of smoking in movies has accelerated in the past decade and that kids exposed to more movie smoking have a significantly higher rate of initiating smoking.

Teen smoking is a big deal to me because it's the gateway to drug use. Teens who smoke cigarettes are fourteen times more likely to try marijuana than those who never use tobacco, according to a study conducted by the American Legacy Foundation and Columbia University's National Center on Addiction and Substance Abuse. Researchers said one reason smokers migrate easily to marijuana is because tobacco use conditions the lungs to accept foreign substances.

I think the most effective way to keep your kids from smoking is to never smoke yourself—or, if you are now a smoker, to stop! Get help from your doctor or pastor, or from friends who have quit. The next most effective way to prevent your kids from smoking is to let them know (1) you expect them not to smoke and (2) there will be consequences if they choose this self-destructive behavior.

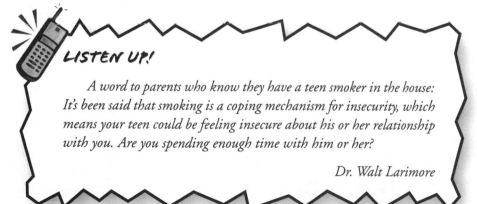

LISTEN UP!

A word to parents who know they have a teen smoker in the house: It's been said that smoking is a coping mechanism for insecurity, which means your teen could be feeling insecure about his or her relationship with you. Are you spending enough time with him or her?

Dr. Walt Larimore

CAN YOUR TEEN COUNT ON YOU?

Many parents assume their teens will ignore them, but that's simply not true. Teens look for guidance in their lives—and their parents are the ones they look to most. Conversely, among teens who get in trouble with drugs or alcohol, surveys are showing that their parents haven't talked with them regularly about the dangers of drug use or drinking. I'll cover the importance of the parent-teen relationship in greater detail in chapter 11 (see pages 224–27).

In the next chapter we'll move on to another important topic in assessing the condition of your teen's emotional wheel—the implications of having a television and Internet access in your teen's bedroom.

Chapter 10

HOME CHANNEL NETWORK

Another aspect of your teen's emotional wheel that must be addressed is the role of media in his or her life and how it affects the way he or she views the world. The mostly harmful influence of Hollywood movies, DVD and video rentals, popular music, entertainment magazines, and surfing the Internet on adolescent emotions cannot be underestimated.

I'll boil it all down to two simple questions:

- ❖ Does your teen have a TV in his or her bedroom?
- ❖ Does your teen have a computer with Internet access in his or her bedroom?

If you answer yes to either of these questions, then you've opened up a pipeline into their bedrooms that can have a dramatically negative effect on their emotional health. Sure, the content can be uplifting at times (*Masterpiece Theatre* and websites for the Louvre Museum), but more often, what flows through the TV cable and the broadband connections could have been pumped in from a sewage treatment plant. Whether used for good or for bad, television and Internet access are powerful media sources that teens find virtually impossible to ignore.

Today's generation of young people is the first to grow up wired to the global village with cell phones and instant Internet access. Looking at it another way, it took forty-five years for electricity to go mainstream, twenty-two years for radio to achieve general acceptance, sixteen years for personal computers to show up in homes, thirteen years for mobile phones to reach ubiquity, and just seven years for the World Wide Web to change the way we communicate. These changes are happening so fast you may not have noticed how the new media has been adopted by the teen world. From tapping "CULTR" (see you later) messages on their cell phones to participating in the free-for-all Instant Messaging chats online, teens hop from one form of media to another all day long—and much of the night too.

I know you can't stand in the way of progress, and I leverage these media myself. I syndicated a sixty-second feature called "Focus on Your Family's Health" that was broadcast on dozens of radio and TV stations, and you've probably noticed I tout my website often in this book. I have nothing against TV or the Internet—just with what folks access on them.

If your teen has a TV or online access in his or her bedroom, you may have no idea what he or she is looking at behind closed doors. These TV shows and web pages may be damaging his or her emotional, relational, and even spiritual health, and spending too much time in front of the TV or a computer screen can have a negative effect on his or her physical health. With that in mind, you can help your teen learn to discern what's good, what's bad, and what's ugly.

Let's take a closer look at these 800-pound media gorillas stalking about the bedroom.

THE TELEVISION

The next time you visit someone's house for the first time, count the number of TVs they have. (The record I've seen is ten.) The U.S. household average is 2.24 sets. You'll find "idiot boxes" (that's what Dad used to call them) in living rooms, family rooms, kitchens, master bedrooms, basement rec rooms, kids' bedrooms, bathrooms—even garages. The Larimore household has been pretty average: we fluctuated between two and three TVs in our home while Kate and Scott were in the teen years.

Those TVs have a way of staying on for long periods of time. ACNielsen, the polling company employed by major networks and cable companies to measure viewership ratings, says that in U.S. homes, the TV is on for an average of six hours and forty-seven minutes during the day. Granted, not everyone's eyes are glued to the tube every single second. Sometimes, the TV is nothing more than background noise while preparing dinner, taking showers, and cleaning up around the house. But most surveys I've seen show that American families are watching at least *four* of those hours each day, while a Harris Interactive Poll from 2003 revealed that teens watch TV about half that much—approximately two hours daily. (If this sounds low, it's because they are spending *more* time on the Internet each day, which I'll cover later.)

I, along with other members of the American medical community, feel that heavy television viewing has serious health risks. Watching TV is a passive and sedentary pastime. You're not firing many synapses in the brain. I was intrigued to read a functional MRI scan study that showed a difference in brain activity between teens watching TV and teens playing board games or participating in robust discussions. The latter activities showed the brain continuing to develop, while slackjawed TV watchers barely registered a blip on the scan study.

Nor are your teens burning many calories working the remote. Instead of using that time to exercise, they're very likely setting themselves up to become tomorrow's next generation of couch potatoes. According to a report in the *American Journal of Public Health*, an adult who watches three hours of TV is far more likely to be obese than an adult who watches less than one hour. As your teens sprawl on the couch, they are targeted by fast-food restaurants and junk-food manufacturers whose thirty-second spots entice them to eat their high-calorie, high-fat, and high-salt foods and drink their sugar-heavy drinks.

Not only can TV make many teens fat (some say just by looking at those ads), it can prompt some of them to become too thin. Three-quarters of American women believe they are too fat, an image issue aggravated by viewing young, attractive, and rail-thin young women in show after show after show. In my years of medical practice, I've seen that this pressure can lead to bulimia and anorexia.

Teens often imitate what they see on TV and in videos, which can present a health hazard. Boys set themselves on fire and lodged toy cars in their anuses after watching Johnny Knoxville and others perform such moronic stunts in the *Jackass* movie. The Los Angeles Police Department reported a rash of street-racing incidents after *2 Fast 2 Furious* was released in 2003. More than ten years ago, a pickup truck in Pennsylvania hit two teens as they lay on the freeway, leaving one dead and the other seriously injured. The parents said the teens were imitating a scene from the Disney movie *The Program*, which showed people lying in the middle of the street as cars zoomed past—all in an attempt to prove their courage and manhood. Finally, how heavily influenced were Columbine High's Dylan Klebold and Eric Harris by *Natural Born Killers*, which showed the characters played by Woody Harrelson and Juliette Lewis conducting trench coat–style killings in the classroom?

It seems clear Klebold and Harris—like their contemporaries—had to have been influenced in some part by the 40,000 murders and 200,000 acts of violence they witnessed while watching TV as they grew up. I don't know how many murders Scott watched growing up (Kate, the reader in our family, rarely watched TV during her middle school and high school years), but I'm sure it was too many.

For many years, Barb and I had two TVs in the home—the family room and the master bedroom—and we'd routinely invite the kids to plop on our bed just before bedtime. On occasion we'd watch TV together if there was something interesting on. When Scott turned fifteen, he asked whether he could have a TV in his bedroom. He even offered to pay for it. His wasn't an unusual request. These days, more than half of parents report that their children have televisions in their bedrooms. In addition, 42 percent of children ages nine to seventeen have their own cable or satellite television hookups in their bedrooms.

I wasn't aware of these shocking statistics when Scott asked whether he could have his own TV. I said I'd talk about it with Barb and get back to him. Because I wasn't as sensitized to this issue as I am now, I discounted Barb's feelings when she voiced concern about letting him bring a TV into his bedroom. We went back and forth, as married couples often do. Eventually she gave in, and we told Scott he could get a TV, as long he bought it with his own money.

What a mistake! That TV was like a large magnet for Scott, who was sucked into his bedroom about fifteen seconds after he finished his last bite of dessert, and we wouldn't see him again until the next morning. It pulled him away from our family, and we had no idea what he watched. That decision, we would all admit now, was a big mistake for Scott and for our family.

Allowing teens to watch what they want whenever they want is like inviting a total stranger who doesn't share your values to spend a lot of quality time with them. What a lousy parenting move on my part, and I should have listened to Barb's intuition. Certainly with a third television in the home, we were less conversational as a family. I have a sneaking suspicion Scott succumbed to the temptation to catch the Leno and Letterman monologues on school nights, which cut into his sleep time and made him more tired in the morning.

Even though Scott has a good head on his shoulders, there's an awful lot of questionable content to be tempted by. Even the basic channels' prime-time shows revolve around talking about sex, thinking about sex, having sex, and what to do after sex. One study of 450 young people revealed that 66 percent said they watched at least one program a month containing nudity or heavy sexual content! Many of today's sitcoms have story lines about gay characters who've been accepted by everyone but the creepy Christian types.

And how about the local news that comes on the tube at 10:00 or 11:00 p.m.? "If it bleeds, it leads" is the mantra of news directors, but what concerns me more is how local TV can hype a story until you're afraid to step outside of your house at night. UCLA researchers found that television news in Los Angeles skewed viewer perception of actual threats to life and limb, causing unwarranted anxiety over some risks while masking the danger of others. The drumbeat of "the sky is falling" stories—arsenic in the water, bad cops on the beat, juvenile crime—can alter the reality of even the most optimistic person.

You would think more parents would get rid of TV—or at least drag the family TV out to the garage, as I heard of one parent doing, to make it less comfortable to watch. Yet, many parents figure that television is fine as long as it's watched in moderation. The question is how to define moderation. For me, anything beyond one hour on a school night—especially given today's heavy homework loads—moves the needle beyond moderation to "heavy."

FYI . . .

► What's That Movie All About?

It's Friday night at suppertime, and your teen is nagging you to see the latest movie everyone at school is talking about. Or he wants to go over to a friend's house and watch one of the new videos just released at Hollywood Video. What do you do?

Run, don't walk, to my website (www.highlyhealthy.net), where I link you to Focus on the Family's "Plugged In" website, which reviews movies from a faith-based, moral perspective. Once you know what a movie is about, you can make an informed decision. Whether teens are watching movies on video or in first-run theaters, you as the parent must have the final say.

Here are a number of sites where you can read online movie reviews written from a Christian perspective—as well as reviews of TV shows and popular music releases:

❖ *Focus on the Family's Plugged In.* You can reach Plugged In's reviews through www.highlyhealthy.net, or go directly to PluggedInMag .org. Access is free.

❖ *Preview Family Movie and TV Review Online.* For $24 a year, you gain access to the latest reviews. It's worth checking out at www .previewonline.org.

❖ *Screenit.com*. While not an overtly Christian website, their movie reviews appear to come from a moral worldview. You find out what's in the movies and read thoughtful reviews. Access is free.

❖ *MovieGuide*. I have more to say about Ted Baehr's movie review service below, but it's on the Web at www.movie guide.org. Cost is a suggested donation of $40 per year.

This is just a small sample of what's available. You can also type "Christian movie reviews" into your favorite search engine and be handsomely rewarded.

If you're not Internet savvy, you may want to subscribe to *MovieGuide* newsletter. Ted Baehr, the publisher, speaks to parents and teens around the country, and he believes Christian kids are seeing the bad PG-13 and R movies in the same numbers as unchurched kids. He says Hollywood has been targeting the "baby boomlet" children—the 77 million born between 1979 to 1989—for years. As these boomlet kids entered the teen years (where your kids are), Hollywood stepped up its output of PG-13 films, which range from the *Dumb and Dumber* franchise to horny teen films like *American Pie* and its ilk.

Bottom line: you need to know what the movie is about in order to make an informed decision. I suggest you read about the film on one of the websites I've described and ask your teens what they think. Does this movie meet the family standard? Could the whole family watch the film or video together? If not, find something else.

Warning: Health Hazards Ahead

Teens who watch TV several hours a day are participating in an activity that can harm their health.

❖ *Teens who watch too much TV aren't as creative.* Referred to by some as a "plug-in drug," television has a way of narcotizing viewers, especially teens, into noninteractive passivity. Studies have shown that those who are obsessed by TV are less creative and more passive.

❖ *Teens who watch TV don't exercise much more than their eyelids.* I've already mentioned the strong relationship between the amount of time teens spend in front of the television and being overweight. One researcher found that "children watching TV tend to burn fewer calories per minute—not only fewer than those engaged in active play, but also fewer than those who are reading or 'doing nothing'—in fact, almost as few as children who are sleeping." The heavier a teen, the more grave the effect. For teens of normal weight, "TV-watching triggered a 12 percent [metabolic] drop . . . the metabolic rates of obese children fell an average 16 percent." Thankfully, these effects are reversible. Some studies have shown that overweight children can lose weight simply by decreasing their television viewing.

❖ *Television violence desensitizes impressionable minds and hearts.* TV dramas keep upping the violence ante because they think they have to outdo the other top-rated shows by broadcasting more mayhem and destruction. The crime scene investigation shows are replete with homicide detectives investigating gruesome deaths. Viewers will often be shown realistic-looking bullet wounds (take it from a doctor— they look real) and macabre killings, such as throats being garroted.

❖ *Television decreases interaction within the family.* As a family's television time increases, family interaction decreases, and relating with their families is the heart's desire of a majority of today's teens. In a nationwide, ethnically balanced survey of 750 ten- to sixteen-year-olds, "Three-quarters said that if they had a choice between watching TV or spending time with their families, they'd opt for family time."

❖ *Teens will not get smarter watching TV.* It seems clear that the more time teens devote to watching TV shows, the poorer their overall school performance and their standardized test scores will be. I agree with the many educators who believe television promotes passive learning and tends to shorten attention spans.

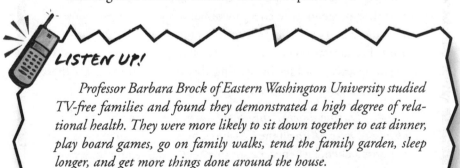

LISTEN UP!

Professor Barbara Brock of Eastern Washington University studied TV-free families and found they demonstrated a high degree of relational health. They were more likely to sit down together to eat dinner, play board games, go on family walks, tend the family garden, sleep longer, and get more things done around the house.

Dr. Walt Larimore

Given all the negative aspects of television, some families have chosen to pull the plug. If TV is a thing of the past in your family, you deserve a parenting award. But if families take strong halfway measures—like having TV-free nights, banning the TV on school nights, or not allowing the TV to be turned on until after dinner—they're doing a great service to their children.

I urge you to pay attention to how often the TV is on in your household and then to take steps to turn it off as much as you can—for their health as well as for yours.

FYI...

▶ Because teens see a lot of unhealthy behavior on TV, they're guaranteed to run into one of "Dr. Walt's Top Six Television Myths" sooner or later:

Myth #1: Promiscuous sex never has any consequences. Many shows and movies—especially those targeted to the teen demographic—show promiscuous sex in the best possible light. Sex is portrayed as something spontaneous, fun, and so right. It's certainly okay to go to bed after you meet in a bar earlier that evening, and anyone who doesn't have "something on the side" is a dweeb. The consequences of promiscuous sex are swept under the sheets. Her getting pregnant? Virtually never happens in TV land. Him getting herpes? Ditto. The potentially lifelong heartbreak after the inevitable breakup? You'll never see it—and it's not only a bad message for your teen, but a completely unrealistic one. I've seen the real-life consequences of promiscuous sex—the shock and tears of a high school girl who learns she's pregnant; the college woman whose boyfriend gave her one or more nasty sexually transmitted infections; the guy with gonorrhea. Premarital pregnancy is a life-changing event that eclipses everything except a life-threatening disease, but no one on these shows seems to worry about it happening.

Myth #2: During a police investigation, it is required to visit a strip club at least once. With all the CSI-type shows on the tube these days, it's almost a cliché: whenever cops investigate the seamy underworld of crime, they invariably end up looking for the bad guys in a strip club. At night. During business hours. In the middle of a show. The next time you flip on one of these shows, watch how the director puts the protagonists in a scene that allows us to see women—and men—in various states of undress at fitness clubs, locker rooms, or strip clubs. (Did I say that before?) Funny, you never see the cops visiting churches on Sunday mornings.

Myth #3: When cars crash, no one gets hurt. Chase scenes are a staple of any Sunday night "Movie of the Week." After bouncing through the streets of San Francisco or burning rubber in Miami, fast and furious drivers either arrive at their appointed destination without a single hair out of place or walking away without a scratch if they've crashed. Of course, the cars usually blow up in a spectacular fireball—but the good guys always get out in time.

Myth #4: One man firing at twenty men has a better chance of killing them than twenty men firing at one man. Gun violence on cop dramas is cartoonish. Bullets fly everywhere and nobody ever gets hurt—until the bad guy gets it just after the last commercial break. Take it from someone who worked in an emergency room in Central Florida and saw his share of gang shootings: when bullets fly through the air, they have a nasty habit of finding the soft flesh of human bodies. Bullets tear flesh and kill people.

Myth #5: A cough is usually the sign of a terminal illness. If you ever watch one of those tearjerker movies on the Lifetime channel, watch out when the lead character has a coughing spell. That person is doomed!

Myth #6: Homosexuality is cool and risk free. Nearly every sitcom features a gay character in today's *Queer Eye for the Straight Guy* world.

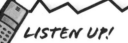

LISTEN UP!

The primary danger of the television lies not so much in the behavior it produces as in the behavior it prevents: the talks, the games, the family festivities and arguments through which character is formed.

Urie Bronfenbrenner, child development expert

ONLINE ALL THE TIME

If you're looking for evidence that teens have embraced the Internet, look no further than a recent Harris Interactive Poll showing that teens spend more time online than watching television. According to Harris, young people spend 16.7 hours online in an average week, compared to 13.6 hours watching TV and 12 hours listening to the radio. Phones took a 7.7 hour chunk out of their lives weekly.   And the TV networks wonder why their market share keeps shrinking.

The Internet, like any media form, can be used for good or for bad. Just as it didn't take long for some people to realize that magazines would be a good place to publish photos of naked women, it didn't take long for "adult" content to arrive on the Internet. Some say porn and the Internet were born for each other. Nobody can see you—as long as you're behind closed doors.

In the old days—the 1950s and 1960s when I was growing up—you had to drive your car or take a bus to a seedy part of town to watch an X-rated movie or buy glossy magazines depicting naked couples performing various sex acts. There was a certain embarrassment about sneaking around in a red-light district with your coat pulled up over your collar. The blush factor faded, however, with the advent of videocassettes, which could be mailed to your home or rented from the video store with the adult section in the back. But renting X-rated videos sounds like a nuisance now compared to the convenience and availability of the myriad of free sites on the Internet. The invention of the World Wide Web and easy access to it via a home computer have ushered in a seismic change in the way pornography is available to your teen.

Internet porn is so widespread that it's almost impossible for your teen not to run into it if he or she is doing homework or research online. The way various search engines are set up, your teen types in a few keywords, and up pops hundreds of thousands of links to various websites that match their search. While many are legitimate, some are porn sites with domain names that include one or more of these key words. For example, an innocent search for "ladybugs" may land your teen at a filthy porn site; researching for a book report on Louisa May Alcott's *Little Women* may lead your teen to a site featuring photos of naked little women. Even if your teens are the most careful Google searchers in history, it's amazing how porn sites discover their email addresses and spam them with porn. It happens to me too frequently.

For teens who type Web addresses into the browser, pornographers will "cybersquat" on other domain names, hoping that your youngster makes a keyboard mistake. Let's say your son is doing a report on the White House or is required to send an email to the president. The official website, he learned in school, is www.whitehouse.gov. What would happen if he absentmindedly typed in www.whitehouse.com? He'd be escorted to a porn site that boasts of being voted "#1 adult website."

And if that isn't bad enough, online chat rooms are forums for people to pretend to be anyone they want to be. Men can join a teen girls' chat forum, and your daughter has no way of knowing who's conversing through typed messages. Among the saddest newspaper reports are those stories of a fourteen-year-old going to a mall to meet someone she met on the Internet and either never being heard from again or being taken to a hotel room by a molester.

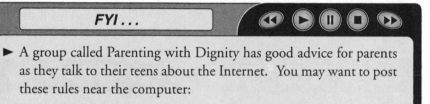

> **FYI...**

▶ A group called Parenting with Dignity has good advice for parents as they talk to their teens about the Internet. You may want to post these rules near the computer:

❖ Tell your teens to always use a screen name. They should never reveal their real name, school, age, phone number, or home address—not even the city or state—when they are online. There are too many predators out there.

❖ Tell your teens to let you know if they receive frightening or upsetting emails.

❖ Tell your teens never to send their photographs over the Internet.

❖ Tell your teens about the dangers of meeting someone they've communicated with in a chat room. The reality is, teens have been kidnapped, raped, and killed after doing this.

❖ Tell your teens to be leery of chat rooms. Instant Messaging with friends is one thing, but you can't accept at face value what a person says in a chat room.

Monitoring Techniques

I highly recommend that parents purchase blocking software and limit Internet access to computers in a public area. Teens surfing the Web in the family room or in a cubbyhole off the kitchen are much less likely to click on a porn site if the opportunity is there for you to easily peek over their shoulders.

The technology is also available to monitor the Internet sites they click on by checking their cookie files, browser caches, and history lists. You can do a search for .jpg or .gif files to find downloaded pictures. (If you don't know how, ask a friend—or your teen—to show you. That's what I did with Scott. He walked me through it, and then I took it a step further and asked him if we could be accountability partners. A couple of times a week, we'd look at each other's Internet history to keep us honest. He was keeping an eye out for me, and I was watching out for him.)

With that background, you can understand how Barb and I felt when my wife found a picture of a naked woman printed from Scott's computer. When she showed him the picture and asked him what was going on, Scott turned white. "It wasn't me!" he pleaded. "It must have been Kyle" (his pal at the time).

"Whether it was Kyle or not, you are responsible when that computer is turned on," Barb informed him.

Check It Out!

▶ Blocking software—Cyber Patrol, Net Nanny, and SurfWatch, for example—makes it more difficult for teens to venture into inappropriate areas. The Christian Medical Association recommends Bsafe Online blocking software. These filtering solutions aren't perfect, however, and porn sites employ clever technicians to figure out ways to get around blocking software. Learn more about Internet filtering on my website (www.highlyhealthy.net), where you'll be able to access the Parenting with Dignity and FilterReview.com websites.

I used that incident to provide a teaching moment. We went out to a restaurant, and I told him we had a great opportunity to talk about the things he was putting into his mind. "Women are relational," I said. "They are about touching and feeling and holding hands. That's very important to a woman's sexuality. For us guys, it's all visual. We see a scantily clad girl and *boom*. We get turned on real quick by what we see."

Scott nodded as he listened. I asked him some questions about the picture. "What color was her hair?" "What color were her eyes?" "What position was she sitting in?"

When Scott didn't have good answers, I said, "That's what I'm talking about. You remember seeing certain parts of her body, and those images will stay with you for the rest of your life. When you're in your marriage bed, that picture may come back to you."

I told Scott I still remembered the first time I saw pictures of naked women. It was back in ninth grade when I opened my locker at school. Lockers didn't have locks in those days, and someone had left a magazine—the latest issue of *Nudist Association of America*. Naturally, I was curious as to its contents, so I flipped open to the centerfold—yes, even the *Nudist Association of America* had a centerfold—which pictured a nubile Native American girl stepping into a gleaming swimming pool and showing full frontal nudity. It was the first picture I'd ever seen of a woman without her clothes on, and I still remember it like it was yesterday.

"You want your mind on your wife when you're with her, not an imprint of some picture you've seen," I said to Scott. "If you build a library of those images, they'll be waiting for you every time you have sex with your wife. Yes, God can erase memories, and yes, God can help us forget things, but that's the risk you take."

Scott made a commitment not to look at stuff he shouldn't on the Internet, and I know he's worked hard to maintain that commitment.

FYI...

► The Golden Chain

Another insidious aspect to television watching and long hours on the Internet is the way it cuts into teens' bedtime hours. Trust me on this: teens who don't get enough sleep aren't highly healthy. English playwright Thomas Dekker was aware of the importance of sleep: "Sleep is the golden chain that ties health and our bodies together."

I think it's accurate to say most teens are out the door between 7:00 and 7:30 in the morning during the school year. If your teens have to leave by 7:15, it probably means reveille at 6:15. Back up nine hours, and they should be tucked in by 9:15 at night. Yes, you read me right. Medical research shows that teens need nine hours of sleep a night; any less, and they have trouble getting up in the morning, concentrating on their schoolwork, and performing well in sports.

Sleep, and lots of it, keeps teens highly healthy because restful sleep releases a growth hormone that helps tissues grow properly, form red blood cells that deliver oxygen to their bodies and brains, and promotes healthy bone growth. Sleep is a basic necessity of life, something as fundamental to your teen's health as air, food, and water. Teens who get nine hours of sleep a night wake up feeling refreshed, revitalized, and ready to listen in the classroom. A rested body helps them think more clearly throughout the day—and act less cranky with you! Tired kids get lower grades, don't perform as well in sports, and have more emotional problems than youngsters who get adequate rest.

Parents need a wake-up call about the importance of sleep. Only 14 percent of Americans, according to a national survey by the National Sleep Foundation, have even a vague notion about the need for sleep and the consequences of sleep deprivation. In 1998 sleep deprivation resulted in 37 percent of adults reporting they were so sleepy during the day that it interfered with their activities. And sleepy adults usually mean sleepy kids. In a 1999 survey, 60 percent of children under the age of eighteen complained of feeling tired during the day, and 15 percent of teens admitted to falling asleep at school.

What, then, can be done about the sleep gap for your teen? The answer seems obvious: Help him or her get more sleep! Here are two things I'd encourage you to do:

1. *Start working your teen toward lights out at 9:15 to 9:30 p.m.* You'll probably have to push to get homework done, showers taken, teeth brushed, and clothes laid out long before lights out. The goal of an early bedtime should spur your teen to get schoolwork done and to keep away from the TV. It's not the time for a caffeinated soft drink or for IMing their friends on the Internet, which will only get them wound up.

2. *Model good sleep habits for your teen.* It doesn't do any good to round up the herd for a 9:30 p.m. lights out if you're not getting to bed shortly thereafter. Barb and I tried to be in bed no later than 10:00 on school nights. I was usually up at 5:30 a.m. for my quiet time, and family breakfast started at 6:15. I had to be out the door by 7:00 a.m. to begin hospital rounds. If your family has had poor sleeping habits, don't try to change them

overnight. If you try to change family routines too quickly, you're doomed to failure. Set reasonable goals. If your teen has been going to bed at 11:30 and getting seven hours, shoot for 11:00 p.m. and seven-and-a-half hours. When he or she sees the benefit of getting more rest, you should see increased cooperation.

In our next chapter, we'll begin our discussion of the relational wheel with some observations about the strong link between your family's health and the health of your teens. What can you as a mom and dad do to build a strong foundation for nurturing a highly healthy teen? What if your family is dysfunctional? What if you're a single parent? What if you live in a blended family? What steps can you take to improve your family's emotional and relational health? These are some of the practical questions we'll tackle.

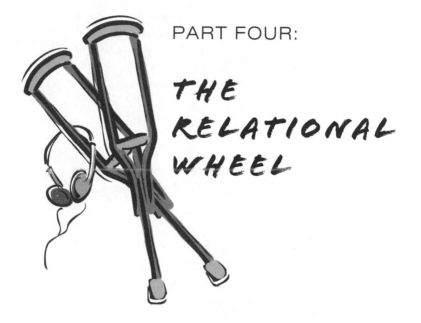

PART FOUR:

THE
RELATIONAL
WHEEL

Chapter 11

FAMILY MATTERS

My wife, Barb, and I have known each other for a long time. We first met in kindergarten. Our families—even our fathers' occupations—were mirror images of each other. Our dads taught at a nearby university and made their families a priority. They married well-educated women who set aside their careers to each raise four children. Our parents practiced strict discipline and maintained high expectations for us. We were required to eat breakfast and supper with the family as much as possible. We took vacations and developed wonderful holiday traditions that often involved the extended family—aunts, uncles, cousins, and grandparents.

Looking back, Barb and I can confidently say we were raised in nurturing families, although at the time we didn't fully understand what a blessing it was. We never heard our parents threaten to divorce each other; the *D* word simply wasn't part of their vocabulary. They were committed to staying together—and keeping the family together—for the long haul.

There's no doubt our solid upbringing provided the foundation for each of us to become a healthy teen. Our parents' commitment to family and marriage provided a strong example for Barb and me. When I asked her to marry me toward the end of our college careers, we looked forward to living near our families and raising a family.

Many young people today don't have the same confidence Barb and I had because they haven't grown up in two-parent "intact" homes like we did. The most recent U.S. census in the year 2000 confirms what many social commentators have observed for years: the institution of marriage is unraveling. The effect of this trend, which began in the 1960s, portends more and more highly unhealthy children and teens. The facts speak for themselves:

❖ For the first time in our nation's history, traditional nuclear families dropped below 25 percent of households.

❖ Thirty-three percent of all babies were born to unmarried women, compared to only 3.8 percent in 1940. In the African-American community, nearly 70 percent of babies were born to single moms.

❖ With a divorce rate of more than 50 percent, more than a million children experience the pain of their parents' divorce each year.

❖ About half of the children in our country spend at least part of their childhood in single-parent, grandparent, foster-parent, or cohabiting-parent homes.

❖ More than 3.3 million children lived with an unmarried parent and the parent's cohabiting partner. Cohabitation now affects three children for every one child affected by divorce.

FAMILY HEALTH TRENDS

These kinds of statistics aren't so easy to sweep under the rug when you consider what our society could look like when today's teens reach their twenties and thirties. "If the family trends of recent decades are extended into the future," writes distinguished Rutgers sociologist Dr. David Popenoe, "the result will not only be growing uncertainty within marriage, but the gradual elimination of marriage in favor of casual liaisons oriented to adult expressiveness and self-fulfillment. The problem with this scenario is that children will be harmed."

I wholeheartedly agree. Today's teen generation is perhaps the first in Western civilization to have several "moms" or "dads," perhaps six or eight "grandparents," and dozens of half siblings or stepsiblings. When teens are rotated through an array of living arrangements, houses, and communities, it's not good for their physical, emotional, and relational health.

The link between the health of a family and the health of its children is undeniable. Scientific research examining the demise of traditional marriages—the lifelong, legal, physical, emotional, social, and spiritual union of one man and one woman—is revealing the devastating effects this demise can have on the health of our teens.

Here's a finding that arched my eyebrow: parental divorce is estimated to increase a teen's risk of developing health problems by 50 percent. The bottom line is that children of divorced, never married, blended, same-sex, or cohabiting parents face higher health risks and are likely to suffer emotionally, academically, and economically. Social researchers believe that teens born into or adopted by first-time married partners do significantly better in all measures of health than children growing up in any other family category.

Common sense would tell any parent that family relationships—as designed by God—are critical. If you are married and the parent of your children, I salute you. The following research is meant to encourage you to continue working on the health of your marriage and to stay with your spouse for the long haul. If you are a single parent, either because you never married or are divorced, you have the toughest parenting assignment of all. I've provided the following information, not to deflate your confidence, but to help you recognize the risks your teens face growing up without both parents in the home—so you can take healthy action now. Here, then, is how teens' health is affected in certain areas:

❖ *Education.* A 2002 study that reviewed more than a hundred other studies published over a twenty-year span found that teens of divorce were twice as likely to drink alcohol, get into drugs, and drop out of high school. When these teens became adults, they were twice as likely to have no degree and to be unemployed.

❖ *Physical Health.* Teens from broken homes are 50 percent more likely to suffer a number of health problems. For example, Dr. Deborah Dawson found that children from disrupted marriages experience greater risk of injury, asthma, headaches, and speech defects than children from intact families.

❖ *Psychological Health.* Children from single-parent families experience more emotional problems than children living with both parents. Children of divorce are especially hard hit. Child psychologist Judith Wallerstein found that children of divorce often experience feelings of rejection, loneliness, anger, and abandonment, as well as a persistent yearning for the absent parent. Five years after the divorce, 37 percent of the children she studied were moderately or severely depressed, which created emotional baggage that often lasted well into the adult years.

❖ *Social Behavior.* Teens of divorced parents are far more likely to become juvenile delinquents, engage in premarital sex, and bear children out of wedlock. Take a survey of any prison population around the country, and you'll find that an overwhelming majority of its residents are products of broken homes.

The verdict is in among social researchers: strong families and marriages are essential to the well-being of children and adolescents. If you are married,

I encourage you to do everything you can to maintain your marriage, because your teens need a father and a mother during this critical period. Even couples who said years later that they "stayed together for the kids" recognized that putting aside their personal happiness for the welfare of their teens was the best decision they had ever made. I believe that a family's stability and predictability, when combined with the ABCD's of emotional health I talked about in chapter 8, are key elements in the emotional and relational lives of highly healthy teens.

FATHERS DO COUNT

If you watch *Hannity & Colmes*—or similar TV shows that bat hot topics back and forth—you'll hear critics of traditional marriage argue that women can raise their children just fine without the fathers. They point to single-parent moms raising good kids against all the odds—genuine success stories. While I tip my hat to these moms who've done a difficult task well, the importance of fathers cannot be discounted.

This lesson was brought home in a poignant way when my daughter, Kate, was a young girl. As I tucked her in one night, she said, "Daddy, can I ask you a question?"

"Yes, pumpkin."

"Will you ever leave us?"

"You mean to go out of town?" I asked.

She thought for a minute, and I saw her eyes flood with tears. "No, Daddy. Will you ever leave us like Janie's daddy left her?"

I gulped as I could see in Kate's face how frightened she was at the prospect of her father abandoning her.

"Honey, I'm committed to your mom, to you, and to Scott for life. I promised my parents and your mommy's parents that I would love your mommy for life. Even more important, I promised God."

I recall this story whenever a media report dismisses the importance of a father in the home. Kate viewed me as part of the whole—someone who supported her mother with love and affirmation and someone who would protect and provide for the family. From the time Kate was six, I took her on dates, so she could see how a man should treat a young woman by opening the restaurant door for her, holding her chair as she seated herself, giving her order first to the wait staff, and engaging in nice conversation.

I'd call Kate from the office and ask her out. She'd check with her mom to be sure it was okay. On the evening of the date, I would exit the house via a side door and walk around to the front door and knock. Our dates were, and still are, a very special part of our lives.

Fathers can have just as much fun with their sons—and teach them a few things about life while they're at it. Playing one-on-one basketball games in the driveway are opportunities for fathers to demonstrate fair play. You call fouls on yourself. You don't hack your opponent. You play hard until the final basket.

Fathers who live with their children are more likely to have close, enduring relationships with their children than those who are physically absent. Fathers who live in another city or state cannot play pickup basketball games with their sons, hash things out over dinner, or be a sounding board as things come up. Sadly, absentee fathers are becoming a big problem. Fatherlessness is a significant epidemic in America—at the beginning of this century 34 percent of all children were living apart from their biological fathers.

Every day in my practice I'd see teens whose fathers were absent. I thought I was pretty good at figuring out whether my young patients had a father in the home until I talked to a school principal. He told me that with just fifteen minutes of interaction, he could predict with 98 percent accuracy whether the teen's father lived at home. The research backs him up. For example, teens living without their biological fathers are twice as likely to drink, smoke, and take drugs, and they are at least two to three times more likely to experience educational, health, emotional, and behavioral problems; to be victims of child abuse; and to engage in criminal behavior than their peers who live with their married parents. In contrast, teens with involved, loving fathers are significantly more likely to do well in school, have healthy self-esteem, exhibit empathy and pro-social behavior, and avoid high-risk behaviors such as drug use, truancy, and criminal activity. The closeness that teens feel to their fathers is one of the most predictable associations with positive outcomes and highly healthy teens.

An analysis of nearly a hundred studies on parent-child relationships by the National Fatherhood Initiative reveals that "father love" is as important as "mother love" in predicting the social, emotional, and cognitive development and functioning of teens and young adults. Another group of researchers found that a loving, nurturing father was as important for a child's happiness, well-being, and social and academic success as a loving, nurturing mother. I've also come across some studies showing that father love is a better predictor than mother love (and sometimes the sole significant predictor) for certain outcomes, including delinquency and conduct problems, substance abuse, and overall mental health and well-being.

Stay the course, Dad. Be there for your kids, and don't let anyone belittle your important role. Your presence is critical to your teen's health.

> **Check It Out!**   ◄◄ ▶ ❚❚ ■ ▶▶
>
> ▶ I'd love to help you become a better father. Go online and take the free hour-long "10 Ways to Be a Better Dad" course. The video clips and notes are great tools to improve your fathering skills. You can find it on my website (www.highlyhealthy.net).

AND MOMS COUNT TOO

Now that our teen years with Kate and Scott are over, Barb and I can look back through the prism of time and observe that we responded to our children differently as they got older, just as they responded to us differently. Kate and I had a tender relationship that reflected her gentle spirit. Scott was a rough-and-tumble teen who required, at times, a stern approach from me. Barb, on the other hand, employed a deft feminine touch. Her intuition could read Scott and his emotions better than I ever could. There were times when Scott responded more quickly to Barb, probably because she is a vessel of mercy and grace. Barb's style of nurturing gave Scott such support that his emotional and relational wheels were always filled with air.

A mother's nurturing, loving support is the air beneath the wings of a teen just starting to soar in life. When teens have this support from their mothers, they feel more confident as they take their first solo flights. Mom's responsibilities can never be successfully delegated, a point underscored by numerous studies showing that teens have a great shot at becoming strong, independent individuals when their mothers have met their needs from a young age. This gives teens the confidence not to run with the crowd, and we all know how vulnerable young people are to go along to get along.

LISTEN UP!

An ounce of mother is worth a pound of priest.

an old Spanish proverb

Moms remain a major influence on their children's health throughout the adolescence years. The mom-teen relationship is especially important when it comes to drug use. Teens find it easier to talk to Mom than Dad about drugs by a large margin—57 percent to 26 percent. Teens who never use marijuana credit Mom more than Dad with their decision not to take a hit by a 29 percent to 13 percent margin. Finally, Mom, take this finding to heart: teens are three times more likely to rely solely on you than their fathers when they face important decisions in life (27 percent to 9 percent).

EVERY FAMILY CAN BECOME MORE HEALTHY

No family is perfect. I haven't met one in my practice, and I certainly didn't return home to one each evening after work. Broken family relationships have been around since Cain clobbered Abel out in the fields, killing his brother. I'm sure his parents, Adam and Eve, were heartbroken to lose a son in such a violent manner. At any rate, our first family quickly became history's first dysfunctional family.

In the next few pages, I'll suggest ways parents of dysfunctional families, as well as single-parent and blended families, can improve their family's emotional and relational health.

Healthy Steps for Dysfunctional Families

Every family hits low spots and encounters times of crisis—a horrible car accident, a mysterious illness, a child's diagnosis of attention deficit/hyperactivity disorder (ADHD). Every family experiences periods of bickering and times of tension. It's just that healthy families tend to have better coping skills and to rebound from their rough patches more quickly than dysfunctional families, where emotional turmoil seems more constant. It's difficult for teens to feel secure in an environment poisoned with sarcasm, a lack of trust, and conditional love based on what they do, not on who they are.

In my experience, most dysfunctional families have one thing in common: one or both parents grew up in a dysfunctional family. The Bible indicates that family dysfunction extends not just to the children but to the third and fourth generations. As dreadful as it sounds, the good news is that the dysfunctional cycle *can* be broken. It may take professional help, however, from a trained pastoral or mental health professional. Many teens growing up in dysfunctional families have developed survival skills for coping with their home situation. They'll need help to see the big picture and guidance to break long-practiced behavioral patterns, which is why I usually prescribe professional counseling.

It can help to spend time with families who seem to have it together. If your son or daughter plays in a soccer or baseball league, your family can get involved in team barbecues and social events. In addition, consider joining a parenting class or a small group at your church. It's amazing how much you can learn from others who are just a few steps ahead of you on the path of life. You may want to plug your teen into an active youth group that meets on a regular basis. Let the group leader or youth pastor know about your family situation so he or she can take an active interest in helping you and your teen. Getting involved in church activities sometimes takes tons of effort and miles of carpooling, but you may well see a positive difference in your teens.

Healthy Steps for Single-Parent Families

I'm amazed when I consider the task a single parent faces—raising children, working a full-time job, maintaining a home, and instilling spiritual values along the way.

Single-parent families usually live with very little money; they are five times as likely to be poor as married-couple families. Against such a backdrop, some ask a boyfriend or girlfriend to live with them, thinking that another adult in the home will help. Having another adult in the home is far different from having a spouse in the home. Because the commitment isn't there, cohabiting women are more likely to experience violence and other conflict in the home. Single-parent moms are far more likely to be beaten, and their teen daughters are at great risk of being sexually abused by a cohabiting male. I always asked about family situations in the examination room, and if I found out the mother was cohabiting, I'd strongly urge her to get out of the situation.

If you are a single parent, you know it's a job that never ends and there's no time to relax. I urge you to build relationships with extended family members—uncles, cousins, and grandparents—who can take one or more of the children for a long weekend or a summer vacation. I urge you to involve your teens in church programs, YMCA programs, Big Brother/Big Sister organizations, and camps that offer safe, positive role models for children of all ages. Get plugged in to your local faith community. The church was instituted by God to be a family for the familyless, and more and more churches have programs that support single parents.

I also recommend reaching out to other single parents for support. Someone who walks or has walked in your shoes can be a willing listener as you cope with the challenges life throws at you. Finding a mentor or a couple of close friends who have succeeded can be enormously helpful. Can you go on evening walks together in the summertime, or visit while the kids play on the swings at the neighborhood park?

Check It Out!

▶ For Internet-active single parents, Focus on the Family hosts a website for single parents. You can link to it at www.highlyhealthy.net. Pastor and speaker Gary Richmond has written a wonderful book called *Successful Single Parenting: Bringing Out the Best in Your Kids*.

Healthy Steps for Blended Families

While blended families are sometimes called "the Brady Bunch," there is no Hollywood ending for many families. Most blended families just don't make it (the remarriage divorce rate is at least 60 percent) because the strain can be so great on the marriage. Blended families are practically guaranteed to clash following the short honeymoon period as two families find themselves living together under one roof. Children (especially teens) tend to regard the new parent as a usurper—sort of a "Mom [or Dad] No. 2."

It can be a challenge to maintain discipline and get everyone on the same page. Each stepparent is naturally more committed to his or her own flesh and blood than to the children of the new spouse. When the inevitable fight occurs between the two sets of children, a stepparent will almost always be partial to his or her children. When these situations occur, it's good-bye to "The Brady Bunch" and hello to "Apocalypse Now." There's no question that such a scenario is highly *un*healthy emotionally, relationally, and even spiritually.

Nevertheless, if you are a parent in a blended family, you can take healthy steps. Keep in mind that some research suggests that a successful connection takes time—usually five to seven years—and doses of professional counseling. It often takes two years or more before a child even begins to accept the stepparent. Meanwhile, much can be done right away:

❖ Establish equitable boundaries for all members of the household and develop traditions to help your two families become a single unit.

❖ Seek mutual respect. As a stepparent, knock before entering a child's bedroom. Children should show respect for the new stepparent and stepsiblings. You as parents must hold the line against embarrassing put-downs or disrespectful attitudes.

❖ Photos from both families should adorn the walls.

❖ Family councils to discuss how the new family is doing should take place several times a month.

❖ When a problem arises that is beyond your understanding, seek the expertise of a family therapist.

By educating yourself, your spouse, and your children and by reading and attending classes on parenting, your chance of success increases dramatically. Seminars, conferences, and retreats especially geared to blended families can help—especially before the blending takes place. Family life and the rearing of teens are too critical, especially for at-risk families, to be attempted on a trial-and-error basis. Check out my website (www.highlyhealthy.net) for helpful resources for your blended family.

No matter what your family situation, raising highly healthy teens takes hard work over many years. We can all continually work on improving the health of our relationships with God, our spouses, and our children. Some of us face more difficult circumstances and greater challenges than others, but every one of us can and must take steps to make our family as emotionally and relationally healthy as possible. Persistent effort today pays huge dividends down the road.

In the next chapter we'll take a closer look at family connections, as well as explore ways to enhance your teen's connections with friends, school and extracurricular activities, and part-time jobs.

Chapter 12

HOW CLEAR IS YOUR TEEN'S CONNECTION?

A ll happy families are alike," wrote Leo Tolstoy in the opening line of *Anna Karenina*, "but each unhappy family is unhappy in its own way." Perhaps Tolstoy was knocking these "happy families" as being too conventional and uninteresting, but nothing could be further from the truth. At the core of what Tolstoy calls "happy families" (and what I call "highly healthy families") are parents and children connected to one another in a way that is mutually satisfying to both generations. On top of this foundation, highly healthy teens tend to be positively connected to the world around them.

We may nod our heads at that simple truth, but in reality all parents have difficulty finding enough time to spend with their teens. And teens need time with their parents to share their problems, successes, hopes, dreams, and disappointments. As hard as this is to do with younger children, the challenge is even greater for parents of teens navigating the choppy waters of adolescence. Yet, for a variety of reasons, most parents assume that their teens need them less as they form strong bonds with friends, schoolmates, and teammates.

How surprised would you be to find out there's a lot of research showing that, instead of pulling away from their parents, most teens prefer to form even closer relationships with their parents? Yes, you read that right! Yet for this to take place, parents must be willing to spend time with their teens— time to listen, time to reason, and time to seek and respect their input. The goal of this difficult but necessary transition is to nurture highly healthy teens who have a strong sense of their individual and unique identity, all the while maintaining a close emotional bond with their parents.

As we discussed the ABCD's of a teen's emotional health in chapter 8, we discovered that a teen's connectedness with his or her parents is characterized by the *quality* of the emotional bond between parent and child and by the degree to which this bond is both *mutual* and *sustained* over time. In such an environment, affirmation, blameless love, connectedness, and discipline result in an emotional and relational climate in which affection, warmth, satisfaction, and trust are balanced with appropriate limits, expectations, and discipline. On this foundation, parents give their children increasing levels of adult responsibility and trust.

Parents and teens who share a high degree of connectedness enjoy spending time together, communicate freely and openly, support and respect one another, share similar values, and have a sense of optimism about the future. The degree of connectedness teens have with their parents has been shown by reams of recent research, or what researchers call a "compelling super-protector" in a family, to protect teens from the many challenges and risks they face in today's toxic culture and world.

CONNECTING IN THE FAMILY

Earlier in the book, I mentioned my friend Edward M. Hallowell, author of *The Childhood Roots of Adult Happiness*. Dr. Hallowell says it well: "Connection—in the form of unconditional love from an adult, usually one or both parents—is the single most important childhood root of adult happiness." Back in chapter 3, I talked about a major decision I had made: to cut back on my patient load two afternoons a week so I could connect with Kate and Scott and spend more time with each of them.

When I initially suggested this to my business partner, I knew I'd have to take a cut in pay. It turned out that 25 percent of my salary was lopped off. Barb was a stay-at-home mom, so my salary was all the money coming into our home. Investing time with my children carried a significant price tag—both monetarily and professionally, but looking back, all I can say is, *What a bargain!* I got to spend two afternoons a week with my children during their growing-up years. During their years in elementary school, I would read to them, take them on walks around the lake, or help them with their homework.

Sharing those experiences was a great way for the kids and me to connect. I remember one time asking Kate whether she'd be willing to help me be more consistent in my spiritual walk. As we batted around the idea, she asked, "Do you think we could have a quiet time together before breakfast?"

Kate knew she (and I!) would have to get up a half hour earlier than normal, but she was eager to "help" Dad. For a number of years, we'd read our Bibles together in the quiet of the dawning day. We also memorized Scripture together—she was a whiz at it while I was a klutz. Her precocious ability to recite Scripture from memory allowed me to compliment her repeatedly—building her self-confidence.

One year we ordered an Adopt-a-Leader kit from the National Day of Prayer website. Kate wanted to pray for twenty leaders, beginning with her school principal, then the school superintendent, our town mayor, the two county commissioners, our state assemblyman, our U.S. congressman, our two state senators, and the U.S. president.

We prayed for our leaders every Friday morning. The Adopt-a-Leader kit came with cards we could send to the leaders to tell them we were praying for them. Among others, Kate sent a card to our new U.S. Congressman, David Weldon, letting him know we were praying for God to give him wisdom as he served the country.

Representative Weldon would send Kate a personal reply each month, thanking her for her prayers and letting her know some specific things she could pray about. They became pen pals. During middle school, our family went to Washington, D.C., and Kate had a special visit with Representative Weldon, where they talked and prayed.

Kate's trip to our nation's capital as a young teen seeded within her a desire to return someday. Following graduation from college, she applied for a White House internship, and she received the nod to become an intern in the speechwriter's office. And guess who was one of the first to invite her to lunch? Congressman Weldon, with whom she had established a long-term prayer relationship.

If you think Representative Weldon was encouraged to know that a teen was praying for him, consider how close Kate and I became when we prayed together. Kate has been challenged by cerebral palsy and doesn't walk well. The teen years could have been very difficult for Kate, but I was blessed to be my daughter's cheerleader and prayer partner. I'm convinced that affirmation (cheering), blameless (unconditional) love, and connectedness (spelled T-I-M-E) provided the foundation for her to become highly healthy.

FYI . . .   ◀◀ ▶ ⏸ ⏹ ▶▶

► *The Family that Dines Together . . . Connects*

Experts tell us that making family meals a priority is more than
worth the effort when our children are in their teen years. The idea
of families sitting down around a dinner table to share meals seems
quaint—something out of an *Ozzie and Harriet* rerun on Nick at
Night. Yet a number of studies report that shared dinner meals are
a major indicator of healthy development for children *and* teens.
Spending quality mealtimes together not only can make your teens
smarter; it can also contribute to their emotional and spiritual
growth. Real bonding happens in those moments when you're
together, sharing the details of your day.

Barb and I considered it vitally important for our family to sit down
at the table for breakfast *and* supper as often as possible. It was a
time to find out what everyone was going to do, or had done, that
day, as well as a time for Barb and me to share our values with Kate
and Scott. It wasn't always easy to eat together. Because of our different schedules, there were weeks when we'd eat only one or two
dinners together, but we worked hard to be at the table together five
times a week. By starting our family dining routine when our children were young, it was easier to stick to it as they grew older and
busier. Kate and Scott looked forward to our family mealtimes as
much as we did. They knew they were being given the full attention
of a mom and dad who were ready to listen and in a mood to discuss whatever they wanted to talk about.

Home family activities are amazingly important to teens. Having a home
your teens feel comfortable in (and enjoy inviting their friends into) builds
family intimacy in ways that increase their self-image. This can mean turning
your basement or family room into a playroom. A pool table, Ping Pong table,
foosball table, PlayStation, or a table where teens can have snacks or play board
games are great accoutrements in a home. These items can sometimes be found
at garage sales for a fraction of their retail price. Let your imagination reign—
we're not talking *House Beautiful* here. Make your teen hangout comfortable.
All you need is some sturdy furniture, plenty of light, a decent rug, and a well-
stocked refrigerator.

Highly healthy families plan great vacations together. An ideal family vacation reduces stress and allows parents and teens to relax together without having to be on the go continually. Camping is an excellent alternative to pricey "fly in" vacations. Time slows down when you pitch a tent in a state or national park. You can get reacquainted with nature as you listen to the wind tickle the branches of tall firs along a glassy lake. There's something magical about sitting around a campfire under the eye of a full moon, swapping stories while making s'mores. Beyond the natural beauty, camping is also a great way to teach teens responsibility. They can help set up the tent, collect firewood, and clean up after dinner.

I realize some families aren't wild about camping. Some turn up their noses at the idea of sleeping in the dirt and using outhouses—which are too far away when you need one and too close when you don't. Others say, "What kind of vacation is that?" If this describes you, then be creative and plan vacations that fall within your budget and play to your interests. Be sure to take some time to consider where your treasure is when it comes to your family. I'd urge you not to make the mistake of skimping on family vacations to keep your teens' wardrobes filled with the latest fashion or to provide them with their own cars. You're sacrificing time for things! And once your teens are out of the house, you can never get that time back.

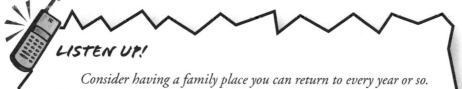

LISTEN UP!

Consider having a family place you can return to every year or so. Maybe it's your favorite ski area, lakeshore resort, dude ranch, or campsite. We have such a place—Santa Rosa Island off the Pensacola coast along the Florida panhandle. A house near the beach has been in the family for more than thirty years, and it's been the site of many treasured family times.

Dr. Walt Larimore

CONNECTING WITH FRIENDS . . . AND MORE FRIENDS

Besides connectedness with parents, highly healthy teens need connectedness with highly healthy friends, activities, and faith communities. As teens gain independence and go out on their own, friendships become more important than ever. Having friends can make a huge difference in their lives—for good or for bad. Just think back to what middle school and high school were like for you. If you had great friends to chat with between classes and eat lunch with, you probably felt life was great. If you felt as though you didn't have a friend in the world, life almost didn't seem worth living. If you ran with a bad crowd, you were likely influenced negatively. As the Bible says, "Do not be misled: Bad company corrupts good character."

Social skills and friendships are huge indicators of teen health and academic success. Teens who are social outcasts can quickly develop what child development experts call a "cycle of rejection." Research shows that teens who experience rejection by their peers are more likely to develop serious emotional, relational, and spiritual difficulties later in life. For example, they don't like themselves, they don't like the relationships they have with others, and they experience the incredible lows of loneliness that lead to depression. You show me teens who are repeatedly rejected by their peers, and I'll show you teens who drop out of school, get involved in juvenile delinquency, and experience their share of mental health problems.

Laura was a quiet but highly creative fifteen-year-old patient of mine. Her mother was concerned about her poor interactions with other teens. She had no friends and she went to weekend parties wearing black clothes and white face makeup—the "Goth" (short for "Gothic") look. I suspected that Laura and her parents weren't connecting at home, and so she needed to connect with her Goth friends instead. Goths often look at themselves as social rejects, unable to fit in with others at school. I recommended that Laura's mom take her to a family counselor.

Several months later, Laura's mom visited me in my house. I asked how Laura was doing. The mother began fidgeting with her hands. "Dr. Larimore," she began, "I'm embarrassed to admit this, but the counselor showed us that Laura's problem was us! We haven't been the parents she needed us to be." She bowed her head and began to weep. Her daughter was an example of someone who needed the close support of her parents, which could help her make friends with more "normal" peers.

Obviously, parents can't accompany their teens to school and help them make friends. However, we must do everything we can to encourage this process. The dinner hour—meal preparation, eating, and cleanup—is a great time to ask open-ended questions such as, "How'd it go at school today? Is anyone being nice? Are you making any friends?"

You can help your teens make friends by encouraging their involvement in groups and activities in which they can excel at something or share a common interest. From a chess club to the French club to a rock-climbing club, you can find something that will appeal to them.

Recent medical research has expanded our knowledge of the importance of friendships on our health. We now know that people who do not regularly enjoy meaningful personal relationships with God or others, or who are in relationships devoid of love or caring, are likely to have dramatically lower levels of health. Lonely teens are at risk to grow up to be lonely adults—and lonely adults are at greater risk for heart attack, heart failure, ulcers, stroke, infectious diseases, mental illness, diabetes, many types of cancer, lung disease, autoimmune disorders, and other life-threatening illnesses. Your teen simply will not become highly healthy without highly healthy friendships.

FYI...

▶ Supporting Your Teen's Friendships

Here are some tips for staying connected as your teen makes friends:

❖ *Get to know your teen's friends.* Before your teen and his or her friends reach driving age, a great way to get to know them is to take them to events. Talking in the car can reveal a lot. Another thing you can do is welcome your teen's friends into your home. Doing this not only provides peace of mind; it allows you to set the rules of conduct and helps you gain a better understanding of what is important to them.

❖ *Get to know the parents of your teen's friends.* It helps to know if other parents' attitudes and approaches to parenting are similar to yours. Knowing the other parents makes it easier to learn where your teen is going, who else is going, what time the activity starts and ends, whether an adult will be present, and how your teen will get to and from the activity. Our teens didn't like it, but Barb and I frequently talked to their friends' parents.

❖ *Help your teen learn that friendships based on looks alone are only skin-deep.* One way to help your teen choose the best sorts of friends is to help them see that good friends have good inner qualities such as loyalty, helpfulness, moral values, and a sense of humor. Talk with your teen about the qualities of their good friends—and praise them for wise choices.

❖ *Provide your teen with unstructured time in a safe place to hang around with friends.* Activities are important, but unstructured time with friends in a safe place lets your teen share ideas and develop important social skills. For example, while with good friends, your teen can learn that good friends are good listeners, that they are helpful and confident (but not overly so), that they are enthusiastic and possess a sense of humor, and that they respect others. Spending time with good friends can also help your teen change some behaviors that make others uncomfortable around him—being too serious or unenthusiastic, too critical of others, or too stubborn.

CONNECTING THROUGH SCHOOL AND EXTRACURRICULAR ACTIVITIES

Many of our teens will participate in an increasing number of activities outside the home as they grow older, which is a healthy thing for maturing adolescents. These activities allow teens to meet, interact, and connect with their peers. Through these activities, teens learn many social skills that will benefit them for life.

There are, however, far more healthy activities in which your teens may want to participate than time allows. Participation in too many activities can be detrimental to their health. Barb and I were careful to help our teens evaluate the activities in which they wanted to participate. We usually limited them to one or two extracurricular activities—especially if the activities involved practice time, training schedules, or time-consuming projects. We wanted our children to learn the qualities of discipline and commitment that can result from participation in extracurricular activities. We also wanted them to have enough time to connect with us, perform well in school, and connect with friends and with members of our church family. These limits may be even more important if your teen wants to work a part-time job.

You can help your teens be highly healthy by helping them consider time commitments, schedules, homework, and other issues before committing to any activity. This is most important at the beginning of the school year when teens are tempted to want to choose several activities to participate in.

Some of the criteria we considered before committing to an activity may be helpful for your family as well:

❖ Barb and I would discuss whether the activity would help our teens learn more about themselves and what they would like to be in the future. We weren't interested in activity just for the sake of activity. We usually had these discussions with Kate and Scott present. We wanted them to hear our line of reasoning and to see us interact and make decisions as husband and wife.

❖ We viewed more favorably those activities that would develop each of our teens' unique talents, gifts, skills, and abilities than we did highly competitive activities.

❖ We evaluated an activity in terms of the cost in money, time, and effort—both for our children and for us as parents.

❖ We compared the cost to the time, money, and energy we had available. In many cases, prior commitments would preclude adding another activity.

❖ All things being equal, we would let Kate and Scott choose their respective activities. We avoided pushing them into activities in which they were not interested or activities that met only our interests or expectations. It was important to let them choose activities based on *their* interests, talents, gifts, time, and desires.

❖ Once Kate and Scott became involved in activities, we viewed our role as being supportive but not pushy.

❖ Once the school year was underway, our job was to watch for warning signs of overcommitment or too much stress—loss of interest in the activity, falling grades, loss of interest in and failure to do homework, physical symptoms (headaches, fatigue, stomach pains), antisocial behavior, or injuries.

I realize these criteria may differ from family to family. But it's essential for your teen's and family's health to carefully evaluate and choose the right balance of activities. Through the years I've seen many parents who didn't do so, and, more often than not, they were going ninety miles an hour—and they were allowing (or even encouraging) their teens to do the same. It almost always resulted in stressed-out parents and children.

In fact, those of us who treat teens are seeing an epidemic of stressed-out adolescents. Many teens in my practice were feeling the pressure of too many responsibilities and too little time. Stress in teens is compounded by overcommitment. To allow (or require) teens to go from school to soccer practice and then violin lessons, followed by a fast-food supper in the car before going to a church social, then to arrive home exhausted and still have homework to do, is a recipe for disaster. Stressed-out teens often suffer from upset stomachs, overeating problems, sleep disturbances, depression, and headaches—and those are just the short-term consequences.

Many parents of my adolescent patients seemed surprised by the amount of homework their teens brought home every afternoon. They didn't account for adequate homework time before they started adding activities such as sports practices, music lessons, club activities, cheerleading practices, band practices, tutoring sessions, study groups, and youth groups. Without question, participation in these activities can be a great experience for many, if not most, teens, but there's no way most highly healthy teens can be involved in more than one or two at a time.

Check It Out!

▶ What if your teen isn't reaching his or her potential in school or struggles to grasp one or more subjects? How do you make the right educational decisions for your teen, given his or her learning style and the options available in your community?

Have you considered a tutor? Have you considered home schooling or enrolling your teen in a charter school, a private school, or a military school? I can direct you to resources that address these critical issues. Check out my website at www.highlyhealthy.net.

When teens become involved in too many activities, the law of diminishing returns comes into play. Instead of feeling excited about the opportunity to excel in a particular area, overscheduled teens simply feel overwhelmed. Parents who desire to nurture highly healthy teens must keep a close eye on their schedule so it doesn't become overloaded. Here are a few common signs that teens are experiencing high levels of stress:

- ❖ grinding or clenching teeth while sleeping, napping, or resting
- ❖ frequent headaches or stomach problems
- ❖ poor appetite or other changes in eating habits
- ❖ fatigue, trouble sleeping, or nightmares
- ❖ compulsive behaviors such as nail biting or lip licking
- ❖ poor concentration

You may be thinking, *OK, you've got my number. What can I do to de-stress my teen?* First and foremost, recognize that it's easier to prevent stress than treat it. If the stress levels are soaring in your home, you may need to cut back on some activities to allow for times of rest and family companionship. Remember, activities don't have to drive the family agenda. Just as it's OK to slow down and relax during a vacation, it's OK—even healthy—to build in some downtime where the family can have fun together and connect in a way that enables parents to show their teens how important and valuable they are.

LISTEN UP!

We need to make sure we're not expecting too much of [our teens]. Evaluate the number of activities they're involved in. If you wonder whether you're overprogramming your kids, you probably are.

Bill McCartney, founder, Promise Keepers

CONNECTING WITH THE WORKADAY WORLD

If your teen is not overscheduled and you feel good about the family connectedness, then part-time work may be another way your teen can develop into a highly healthy adult. After all, he or she does need to learn how to work, and the last I checked, the best way to learn how to work is to work! I know this may be a novel concept in some quarters, but I think it's good for young people to toil in the hot sun or next to a sizzling grill. Honest work teaches young people tenacity, how to handle responsibility, and the value of a dollar. It also teaches teens how to interact with and connect with adults and the adult world in which they'll need to operate. Ideally, your teen's job should be a good match for his or her temperament, gifts, talents, and interests. Your guidance and affirmation can help steer in that direction.

Many teens find that, with a full academic load and involvement in school and extracurricular activities, as well as in club or youth group activities, the opportunity to work during the school year may be pretty limited. It was that way for our teens, who were more available to work in the summer months than during the school year. Barb and I didn't want them to think of summertime as lounge-around, throwaway months but as an opportunity to gain additional education. We steered them toward jobs that would either enhance their values or their job skills. For instance, when Kate started getting asked to babysit, Barb and I thought it'd be good for her to take a babysitting certification course at a local hospital. She was shown how to take care of babies— how to properly hold them, feed them, change their diapers, and place them in their cribs. The course was a great skill-builder for her, and we saw Kate's love for children grow. Having a certificate in her hand helped her land more babysitting jobs in the neighborhood—and even charge a bit more than the going rates. Scott worked the neighborhood in a different way—mowing lawns, clearing out brush, and trimming bushes and hedges. In the Florida summertime, that was backbreaking work. He took a couple of sales jobs when he got older, working at ticket outlets and interacting with the public.

While I can wax poetic about the virtues of hard work, I must temper my comments by pointing out several realities: working more than several hours a week during the school year can negatively affect their grades, keep them from pursuing extracurricular activities that range from sports to drama to chess club, and cause them to skip out on Wednesday night youth group. Therefore, I'd recommend that teens' work during the school year should be very limited—maybe even limited to Saturdays and holiday periods. After all, they already have another important job to do—nurturing healthy connections with friends, working hard in school, and taking part in healthy extracurricular activities, right?

As you implement the principles we've discussed in this chapter, remember this: Research from the fields of social science, public health, medicine, psychology, and education consistently demonstrate that "parent-teen connectedness" (the term used by researchers) is a critical factor for a variety of teen health outcomes, including the prevention of nonmarital sex and pregnancy, STIs, HIV, depression, suicide, alcohol and drug abuse, violent behavior, and poor school performance, just to name a few.

My hope and prayer is that the ideas we've explored will assist you in one of the most important jobs your Creator has ever given you—connecting with your teen as he or she grows into a highly healthy person. And, as you'll see in the next chapter, a strong, mutually comfortable connection with your teen will pay huge dividends as you guide him or her through those turbulent waters of teen sexual activity.

Chapter 13

GETTING ALL HOT
AND BOTHERED

I became Erin's family doctor when she was a young girl. Her pixie-like build—she was a fabulous soccer player—reminded me of gymnast Mary Lou Retton, the Olympic gold medal winner from the 1984 Summer Games. Erin was one of those cute, vivacious, and energetic girls whose thousand-watt smile could light up a room. She came from a great Christian home.

When she turned nine years old, I showed her and her mom the famous "sex video" during an office visit, followed by a discussion of what sex is all about. As is my habit, I spent some time talking about the importance of waiting until marriage to have sex.

Well, beautiful girls grow up to become beautiful young women, and Erin looked stunning when she made an appointment with me toward the end of her junior year of high school. Soccer season was over, so I knew she wasn't seeing me for a routine physical.

I scanned her chart for a moment before saying, "How can I help you, Erin?"

"I'm scared, Dr. Larimore. I did one of those home pregnancy tests, and it came out positive."

That was a bombshell. "I see," I said, trying hard to maintain the non-judgmental tone I normally adopted in these sorts of situations. "You've been sexually active?"

"Yes," Erin answered as she bowed her head. "I've been dating this guy for a couple of years."

"And you'd like me to do a pregnancy test to confirm whether you're pregnant or not," I continued, stating the obvious.

The poor girl nodded, barely able to hold back the tears.

We conducted a pregnancy test, and to everyone's relief, it was negative. Obviously, this reprieve opened the door to talk about the dangers of premarital sex. "Tell me about this fellow you've been dating," I began.

"Well, he's two years older than I am, and he's in the Marine Corps. He pressured me to have sex before he left for boot camp."

"Were you aware of the ramifications?"

"Yes, but he said if I loved him, I would have sex with him. I guess I wanted to show him I loved him."

"You're aware that guys are looking for relationships to have sex?"

Erin nodded.

"And that girls are looking at sex to have a relationship? He wants to mate; you want to marry. Make sense?"

Erin nodded again.

"If you, as a young woman, want to guarantee your relationship will last, don't give the guy sex because (1) once you give him sex, it's *less* likely to become a long-term relationship, and (2) once you make the decision to have sex with him, the question arises: Is he going to have sex with others, even after you're married?"

"I know, but if I didn't have sex with him, he might not have stayed with me."

"Erin, if he had sex with you, the odds are much higher that he *won't* stay with you."

The young woman paused to think. "This presents a problem," she conceded. "What do I do when he comes home for Christmas?"

Now we were getting somewhere.

"You're going to have to make a decision, Erin," I said. "One of the options is deciding to be serious about your faith, that you're going to be serious about your purity, that you're going to choose purity, and that your relationship with God is more important to you than your relationship with any man."

"I think you're right," she said, nodding and smiling. As she left my office, she promised to think about what I said.

On a subsequent visit, Erin told me she had chosen to commit herself to secondary virginity. She stood her ground, and not long after that, the young man asked her to marry him. A year later they were married in a gorgeous military ceremony.

One of the sweet things that happened that evening was a brief interaction I had with the groom during the reception. It was the first time I had met Erin's beau. He thanked me for helping them reestablish their priorities—and for making their relationship a healthy one based on mutual respect and a desire to accept God's boundaries on sexual conduct.

I thanked this honorable young man for his comments, congratulated him on his character, and wished him all the best in whatever God had planned for his future.

STOP IN THE NAME OF LOVE

If only more young couples understood that God's desire that they wait until marriage to have sex is for their physical, emotional, relational, and spiritual benefit.

Take the physical aspect. From a medical standpoint, it's physiologically easy for the body to pick up or transfer a sexually transmitted infection (STI)—and easier for adolescents than at any other time in their lives. During sexual intercourse the erect penis enters the vagina, and during vigorous skin-on-membrane contact, an opening from the male body (the urethra) releases pre-ejaculatory secretions followed by semen, which are then mixed with the woman's cervical fluids in a warm environment. With such close and intimate contact, it's a physical fact that tiny organisms can easily pass from one teen to the other.

Spreading a virus or bacteria from one person to another during sexual activity can happen even without going all the way. If young people who are taught "outercourse" techniques in high school sex ed classes believe that mutual masturbation is the best way to avoid venereal disease—or to avoid becoming pregnant—they could be in for an unpleasant surprise. A surprise weighing six pounds fourteen ounces. Not only that, several STIs can be caught just from touching in the genital area.

When I began in medical practice more than twenty years ago, I was trained to look for a half dozen sexually transmitted infections. In those days, gonorrhea, syphilis, and herpes were the biggies on our history checklist. Today, doctors must be aware of more than three dozen STIs that have been identified by the National Institutes of Health, including:

- ❖ genital warts—fleshy, cauliflower-like adhesions on the penis or around the vaginal area—caused by the human papilloma virus (HPV), which causes cervical cancer in women and has been implicated in penile and prostate cancer in men, and has no current cure

❖ chlamydial infection, the most common of all bacterial STIs, which can cause an abnormal genital discharge and burning sensation when urinating but presents absolutely no symptoms in up to 50 percent of males and 70 percent of females (in women it can silently scar the fallopian tubes and lead to infertility)

❖ trichomoniasis, a bacterial STI that causes an excessive, foamy yellow-green vaginal discharge in women and inflammation of the urethra and glans in men

❖ hepatitis B, an incurable viral infection that produces fever, headaches, muscle aches, loss of appetite, vomiting, and diarrhea, and can be fatal

LISTEN UP!

According to the National Institutes of Health, sexually transmitted infections are infecting more than 13 million new people each year in this country. Nearly two-thirds of all STIs occur in young men and women twenty-five-years old and younger, and the fastest-growing population with new cases of STIs are high schoolers. Social scientists attribute the skyrocketing increases to young people becoming sexually active earlier and marrying later. Translation: sexually mature teens aren't willing to wait.

Dr. Walt Larimore

I've been in the examination room and witnessed the anguish when I've soberly said, "I'm afraid you have a sexually transmitted infection." Many had no clue they could contract an STI so easily. A CDC study released in 2003 showed that 89 percent of girls felt they were at little to no risk of getting an STI. And that's such a shame, because sexually transmitted infections will have a major impact on their physical health. Some STIs can spread into the uterus and fallopian tubes, causing pelvic inflammatory disease (PID), which in turn is a major cause of both infertility and ectopic, or tubal, pregnancy. And as I mentioned earlier in my discussion of pelvic examinations, HPV is now considered to be the leading cause of cervical cancers.

STIs can follow an individual into marriage. Experts estimate that 10 to 15 percent of couples (about 10 million people) have difficulty conceiving. A significant number of these infertility problems arise as a consequence of STIs and thus would have been avoided if both husband and wife had postponed sex until marriage. At least 20 to 30 percent of infertility cases in the United States result from STIs, while in some regions of the developing world the figure is closer to 80 percent. Worst of all, most of the time the STI is unrecognized, asymptomatic, or silent. (Bear in mind, though, that in America most cases of infertility are not related to STIs, and we must be very careful not to jump to conclusions about an infertile couple's "promiscuity.")

Sexually transmitted infections can also attack innocent bystanders—newborns. Various STIs can be passed from a mother to her baby before, during, or after birth, setting off congenital complications that can cause a baby to be permanently disabled or even to die. Early in my medical career, a young teen mom brought in her infant. I hadn't seen the mom during her pregnancy, nor had I delivered the child. She was concerned the child wasn't eating well or growing normally. The child was obviously jaundiced, and my examination revealed that the baby's liver and spleen were enlarged. I diagnosed hepatitis B. Further testing showed the mother was infected too. Sadly, there was no treatment available, and the baby died soon after. It was one of the most tragic cases of my career.

RAISING THE BAR

Parents play a vital role regarding their teen's health in the area of premarital sex. Your ability to communicate the importance of waiting and your expression of unconditional love may well be the impetus they need to stay out of bed, stay out of the backseats of cars, and stay away from groping. Raise the bar as high as you can. Your words and actions should declare that you expect your teens to wait until marriage before having sex. You can tell them, "You may not be able to control your feelings, but you can control your actions."

What can you do to help your teens reach their goals and become highly healthy?

Whenever Possible, Be Home during Nonschool Hours

Spending time with your teen at home can prevent him or her from engaging in premarital sexual activity. You see, teens these days aren't bothering to park at Lover's Lane. Instead, 91 percent of sexually active teens in one study reported they last had sexual intercourse at their family home, their partner's family home, or a friend's house. With their hormones on fire and no adult on duty (and siblings engrossed by TV or homework), teen couples are free to swing for a home run in one of the back bedrooms.

A study by the Urban Institute showed that young boys whose mothers were employed full time had rates of sexual experience 45 percent higher than those of male classmates whose mothers were home when they arrived home from school. The *Journal of Marriage and the Family* reports similar findings for young girls. These studies underscore the importance of a mother or a father being home when their teens are home—especially when they are there with a boyfriend or girlfriend.

FYI . . .

► A research brief filed by The National Campaign to Prevent Teen Pregnancy outlines these implications for parents of teens who are or want to be sexually active:

Adolescents' first sexual experience may very well occur when parents are in the home. Consequently, the primary message to parents is: Whether young people are at home, their partner's home, or the home of a friend, parents should be more aware of their activities. Parents should not be shy about making their presence known around the house. Parents should make sure that a responsible adult is present and paying attention when their children are at the home of a boyfriend/girlfriend or friend. Other research shows that the likelihood of first sexual experience increases with the number of hours teens spend unsupervised. If parents or other responsible adults are not with teenagers, they should take advantage of adult-supervised activities that constructively engage teens.

While parents clearly cannot determine their children's decisions about sex, the quality of their relationships with their children can make a real difference. Overall closeness between parents and their children, shared activities, parental presence in the home, and parental caring and concern are all associated with a reduced risk of early sex and teen pregnancy.

Carefully Monitor When Your Teen Begins Dating

Another vital decision you make is when to allow your teen to start dating. Teens who are given the green light to single date in seventh, eighth, ninth, or tenth grade often adopt a "been there, done that" attitude to boy-girl relationships as they grow older. Going to the school prom with a date isn't very special if they've been going to school dances with dates since sixth grade. A goodnight kiss isn't a big deal if they've been smooching since middle school. Our family rule was that Kate and Scott could start to group date when they turned fifteen but could not single date until they turned seventeen. It's also not wise to allow your daughter to date guys more than one year older than she. A fifteen-year-old freshman girl lacks the emotional maturity or dating experience to rebuff the sexual advances of an eighteen-year-old senior boy.

Research has shown that parents who set moderate, reasonable rules for teens experienced the lowest prevalence of sexual activity with their teens. This included carefully supervising their teens with regard to whom they dated and where they went and setting a reasonable curfew. Parents with very strict discipline and too many rules about dating had *higher* rates of sexual activity among their teens than parents who set more moderate rules. Adolescents who engaged in the most premarital sex lived with parents who set no rules.

FYI... ◀◀ ▶ ❚❚ ■ ▶▶

► *Be Alert to These Risk Factors*

❖ It's so obvious it seems almost silly to mention it, but alcohol and drug use increase the risk of teen sex. Intoxication clouds judgment and weakens resistance to sexual overtures.

❖ If a parent sends the message that teen sex isn't such a big deal, the teen is more likely to have premarital sex. These misguided, permissive parents often say, "Don't do it, but in case you do, use this condom or be sure you're taking a birth control pill." Teens who get this message are likely to act accordingly. I know—I've seen them in my office.

❖ Many parents don't understand that frequent family relocations increase the risk of teen sexual activity. Moving stresses both parents and children, especially if the kids resent the decision. Bonds to social support systems that help prevent sexual activity—such as youth groups—are severed by multiple moves. Loneliness and loss of friendships may lead some teens to use sexual activity as a way to gain social acceptance. These issues should be carefully considered by parents who are pondering a relocation. It may be better to wait until your teen finishes high school, if that's at all an option.

❖ Teens who are in single-parent families run the risk of being sexually active. Parenting is designed to be a team effort, and it is most effective with a husband and wife living under the same roof. The risk for teen sex will naturally increase when one parent is left to do all the protecting and monitoring alone. This increased risk doesn't mean adolescent sex is inevitable in single-parent homes, but it does place an additional responsibility on single moms and dads to send their teens clear, consistent messages about sexuality.

TALKING TO YOUR TEEN

Many parents in my practice who had followed my advice to start talking about sex to their children in early childhood (I give tips in my book *God's Design for the Highly Healthy Child*) felt that by the time their kids were adolescents, they didn't have to talk about sex anymore. Nothing could be further from the truth. The teen years are an even more critical time to talk about sex, so keep up the chatter.

In the preteen and teen years, you and your spouse will have the privilege and responsibility of emphasizing the news that sex is a wonderful gift designed by God to bring new life into existence, to generate a powerful bond between a husband and wife, and to be intensely pleasurable. You can teach your teen that sex is an extraordinary thing that deserves to be treated with great and abiding respect and that God designed "the act of marriage," as author Tim LaHaye calls it, to work best and to be nurtured best between a lawfully wedded couple—one man and one woman. And you can let them know that at the wrong time with the wrong person, sex can bring disappointment, disease, derailed life plans, and lifelong consequences.

Have no doubt, even if your teen doesn't talk to you about sex, he or she is intensely curious about the subject and wants to know the truth. Don't expect to communicate your values in a few lengthy sessions. Brief but potent teachable moments crop up regularly throughout childhood and adolescence. When the tabloids splash some exposé on the front page, or when you hear the news of a pregnancy crisis in another family, take advantage of such powerful teachable moments. You can clearly note that incidents of nonmarital sex are wrong, but be sure to respond with compassion and prayer for the people involved. By doing so, you make it clear you can be approached if anyone at home has a problem. But if your response is, "Don't you ever do something as stupid as that," or "That stupid girl brought such shame to her family," you may block critical communication with your teen in the future. Crisis pregnancy centers find that many of their most painful clients are daughters of the "pillars of the community"—good, moral, upright, churchgoing parents. As these girls head out the door for the abortion clinic, their refrain often goes like this: "I can't tell Mom and Dad; it'll kill them if they found out what I did." And another unborn child dies.

While it's good to state your principles about sex with consistency, conviction, and clarity, your teen must understand he or she can come to you when he or she has problems. If your teen is convinced you'll "kill her" if you find out what she's done, then you'll be the last to find out. But if she knows you are a source of strength when trouble comes, you'll be able to help her contain the damage if she makes an unwise decision. And indirectly, you may show her the attributes of God, who is her ultimate refuge and strength.

If you haven't done so already, plan a special evening or a weekend away from home in which a discussion of the importance of preserving sex for marriage can be the focus. (I recommend that a father share this time with his son, and a mother with her daughter. Some especially close families can accomplish this with both parents present, but the child may feel you're teaming up against him or her.) Some parents use this time to ask their teens to make a covenant with God to remain sexually pure until marriage, and they give their son or daughter a special token—a necklace or ring, for example—to symbolize commitment to an abstinent lifestyle.

LISTEN UP!

Don't give up if your efforts to broach the topic of sex aren't greeted with enthusiasm by your teen. Even when your tone is open and inviting, you may find that a lively conversation is harder to start than a campfire on a cold, windy night. Your thoughts may be expressed honestly, tactfully, and eloquently, but you still may not get rapt attention from your intended audience. Be patient. Don't express frustration, and don't be afraid to try again later. In spite of all appearances, your teen may be hanging on every word.

Dr. Walt Larimore

THE POWER OF YOUR INFLUENCE

The reasons so many teens choose to engage in premarital sex are many and complex. Normal teens—even yours—have intense sexual interests and feelings. They also deeply need love and affirmation. Sadly, our culture practically drowns teens in sexual and seductive messages. Therefore, unless teens live in complete isolation, they will be regularly exposed to sexually provocative material that expresses immoral viewpoints, fires up their sexual desires, and wears down resistance to physical intimacy. What's more, a teen's natural modesty is often dismantled during explicit presentations about sexual matters in the mixed company of a high school classroom.

If you add up these factors and multiply them by the incredible peer pressure they face, it's amazing that half of our teens remain virgins throughout high school. This peer pressure can come from the mistaken notion that "everyone is doing it," although clearly half are *not* doing it. Most teens I cared for kept a mental tally of reasons for and against premarital sex. Their sexual drives, the cultural messages, and peer pressure pulled them toward sex. On the other side of the ledger, the moral standards taught at home and church, combined with medical warnings, weighed in against premarital sexual activity. For most teens, even those who want or intend to abstain until marriage, the decision about having nonmarital sex tends to be based on this internal tally. Therefore, when the moment of truth arrives, the tally may be close— or a landslide in the wrong direction.

This is where your relationship with your teen comes into play. Teens who have a shaky or negative self-concept or who don't experience affirmation, blameless love, connectedness, and high expectations at home are particularly vulnerable to sexual involvement. That's why it's so important to make the effort to have ongoing conversations with your teen about the many compelling reasons to postpone sex until the wedding night.

Fathers particularly need to understand their vital role. A boy who sees his father treat his mother with physical and verbal courtesies and is taught to do so will be more likely to carry this behavior and attitude into his own relationships with women. Girls who are consistently affirmed, unconditionally loved, and treated respectfully by their fathers aren't as likely to search for male affection, which can lead to sexual involvement—and they'll learn to expect appropriate behavior from the other men in their lives.

Teenagers who feel inadequate, incomplete, and unappreciated are more likely to seek comfort in a sexual relationship. But those with a life rich in relationships, in family traditions, activities, interests, and, most of all, in consistent love and affirmation are less likely to embark on a desperate search for fulfillment that can lead to unwise and dangerous sexual decisions.

LISTEN UP!

The home environment makes a difference in the health of American youth. When teens feel connected to their families and when parents are involved in their children's lives, teens are protected.

Robert W. Blum and Peggy Mann Rinehart,
University of Minnesota

THE SEX EDUCATION CURRICULUM

No matter how involved you are in your teens' lives, don't forget other voices are competing with yours for attention, especially from the media they watch and the curriculum they're taught. At the end of the day, it's up to you to counteract the "safe sex" message that penetrates their ears.

If your teens attend a public middle school or high school, do you know what they're being taught about sex? Do you know whether their sex education is part of an abstinence-based curriculum or a comprehensive curriculum?

Abstinence-based curriculum promotes abstinence as the best way to avoid STIs, teen pregnancy, and teen abortion. Abstinence-only programs teach that the standard is a monogamous relationship within the context of marriage and that sex outside of marriage is likely to be psychologically and physically harmful. Teachers do not talk about contraception except to outline their failure rates.

I've seen firsthand that abstinence education works. When I was practicing in Central Florida, my partner, Dr. John Hartman, and I gave pro-abstinence talks in classrooms—from fifth grade to high school. Over the course of time we saw some pretty dramatic changes in the behavior of teens. When we started, the self-reported virginity rate in our county was around 20 percent. By the time I left Florida, the self-reported virginity rate had leaped to 60 percent, which was well above the national average. Sadly, though, there aren't many school administrators who eagerly invite pro-abstinence doctors to air their views in public school classrooms these days.

You may be wondering why there's even an issue about what kind of sex ed to teach, since abstinence works every time it's tried. But those who promote comprehensive sex education say we know kids are going to have sex anyway, so we may as well teach them how to use condoms and other forms of contraception to protect themselves against sexually transmitted infections and to prevent pregnancy. And it even goes beyond that. You have high school classes where kids unroll condoms over bananas and take tests on the best way to masturbate their partners. Don't think it doesn't fuel your teen's motor, which is why I recommend you excuse your children from comprehensive sex education classes in public schools. If Kate and Scott were attending a public school today, Barb and I would probably pull them out of regular sex education classes or closely monitor what was being taught there. We considered it our responsibility to teach our children in this arena of their lives.

There is a silver lining, however. Pressure from pro-family groups and parents during the 1990s and into the first years of the twenty-first century has pushed federal funding for abstinence-only education to record levels. According to a 1999 study undertaken by the Alan Guttmacher Institute, nearly one-fourth of public school sex education teachers taught abstinence as the best way to prevent pregnancy and STIs in 1999, up from a miniscule 2 percent in 1988.

It's interesting that when it comes to health issues, in every area of prevention we tell our teens, "Just don't do it!" Yet on the issue of conveying the message of sexual abstinence to teens, doctors seem to lose their nerve in the examination room. As both sides of the culture war bicker about the best message to teach our teens, I emphasize that the billions of dollars spent on the safe-sex curriculum since the 1970s hasn't worked. It wasn't until abstinence-only education caught on in the last decade that we've seen a drop in high school students engaging in sexual activity. According to a 2003 CDC survey, nearly 47 percent of high school students (grades nine through twelve) reported ever having had sexual intercourse, down from 54 percent in 1991.

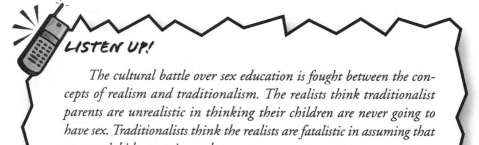

LISTEN UP!

The cultural battle over sex education is fought between the concepts of realism and traditionalism. The realists think traditionalist parents are unrealistic in thinking their children are never going to have sex. Traditionalists think the realists are fatalistic in assuming that everyone's kids are going to have sex.

Brent Bozell, president of the Media Research Center

A CHAT WITH THE DOCTOR

When I lived in Florida, I worked at a faith-based family practice. Our doctors chose not to prescribe birth control pills or hand out condoms like M&M's to unmarried patients. Nor did we do abortion referrals. Nonetheless, I saw my share of young women like Erin who had been sexually active, and I treated my share of teens—male and female—for a variety of STIs. At such moments I saw the need to intervene—to talk to these teens about the dangers of premarital sex and the benefits of postponing sexual activity until marriage. On other occasions, parents would ask me to "have a talk" with their son or daughter.

As Lucy of *Peanuts* fame would say, "The doctor is in," and if I were to sit down with your teen, I'd say something like this. (Feel free to read these pages to your teen or adapt what you've read here to share with him or her the next time the topic of sex comes up.)

Hi, Jimmy. How are you doing today? Listen, I'd like to talk with you about something that'll have a huge impact on your physical, emotional, relational, and spiritual health. It's called premarital sexual activity.

According to the statistics, you have a fifty-fifty chance of having sex before you graduate from high school, and by the time you marry, you'll definitely be in the minority of those who wanted to wait until their wedding night to be sexually active, if that's what you choose to do.

I want to urge you to wait, Jimmy. It's the best health care decision you can make. You'll protect yourself from the possibility of becoming a parent before you are mature enough or financially able to support and raise a child. You'll protect yourself from a variety of sexually transmitted infections. You'll protect yourself from making sexual comparisons when and if you marry. And you'll be doing what God asks us to do in the Bible.

Sexual intercourse creates the most intimate bond a man and a woman can experience. Because it's such an indelible emotional event, past sexual experiences pop up in the mind, kind of like those pesky whack-a-weasels you see at the arcade. The mind, which is the body's most sensitive organ, has a way of recalling memories like they happened yesterday.

One of the biggest negatives of premarital sexual activity is the way it drags past experiences into the marital bedroom. It's easy to play the comparison game because memories of past sexual experiences can flood the senses during arousal and then climb to a peak. Guys can't help but compare the sexual performance of one female against another, or what her body looked like naked compared to another woman he saw naked. Guys will replay these scenes hundreds of times in their minds, and this can't be good for the long-term sexual health of a marriage relationship.

I'm sure you're feeling great pressure to engage in premarital sex—especially because of all the movies and TV shows and commercials that show young people having tons of sex. The problem is they don't show reality. You never see these couples worrying about her becoming pregnant or whether they picked up a sexually transmitted infection. You don't see them getting blood tests in a doctor's office. You never see them crying their eyes out because their boyfriend or girlfriend dumped them to have sex with someone else.

Now that you're growing up and becoming more independent, you may have some opportunities to engage in premarital sex. You're going to have to make a choice today not to put yourself in situations where it would be easy to yield to sexual temptation. You should think about taking precautions, like going out on double dates or making sure you're never home alone with that special person in your life. You should tell the person you have a relationship with what your standards are—how far you're willing to go, how far is too far. I'd say that anything beyond kissing is putting you at risk for going further.

Some adults may wring their hands and say, "They're going to do it anyway," and they'll come to you and hold out a jar of condoms, and they'll tell you to take a few. Don't listen to them! You have the rest of your life ahead of you, and waiting is definitely something worth fighting for. Maybe you'll feel the urges are too great sometimes, but you'll survive just fine by postponing sex until you're married.

First Corinthians 13 describes love as being patient and kind, not envious or self-seeking. The fact that love should be patient is an important lesson when it comes to premarital sex. If you really love someone, you'll be willing to wait to share such a precious gift. If you and your future spouse wait for each other, you'll open an amazing present. My wife and I waited for each other until our wedding night, and it's the best thing we could have done for our relationship. We had built up trust because we both knew we weren't bringing past partners to bed with us, nor were we bringing a sexually transmitted infection into our relationship.

God tells us repeatedly that we need to keep ourselves sexually pure and not open the gift of sex until we're married. In fact, most New Testament books have a verse that shows how important it is to God that we avoid sexual immorality. Acts 15:29 says we should abstain from sexual immorality. Galatians 5:19 says the acts of the sinful nature are obvious—sexual immorality and sexual impurity. Ephesians 5:3 says there shouldn't even be a hint of sexual immorality in our lives. First Corinthians 6:13 reminds us that the body is meant for the Lord—not sexual immorality. Did you hear the common phrase in all these? *Sexual immorality.* What God is saying is that sexual activity outside of marriage is sexual immorality.

God has his reasons for forbidding premarital sex. He knows that teens who engage in premarital sex have a tragic way of becoming parents. The way it is in Western culture, you're a minor until you turn eighteen. Right now, you don't have the education or the job skills to command more than a minimum-wage salary. You can't support a family at this time.

It's worth it to keep yourself pure for that special person God has waiting for you. The Lord designed sex his way for a good reason, and plenty of people who disregarded his plan would tell you how much they regretted giving their virginity away. I can assure you how special it will be to give your spouse something that you haven't shared with anyone else before.

Finally, I'll leave you with this thought. Between now and the time you get married, you'll probably go on a few dates. Some will be casual, and some won't. Either way, you'll likely be spending time with someone you won't end up marrying. You should treat that person with respect and honor, the same way you hope somebody else is treating your future spouse, wherever that person may be.

My passion for helping teens wait for sex until marriage comes out of a context of having been down in the trenches, seeing thousands of teen patients in my office over the years. Some have jumped the gun and had premarital sex. Some contracted an STI; others became pregnant. It's heartbreaking. But there's a message of hope that can arise out of the ashes. If you asked me to talk to your teen son or daughter who's been sexually active, I'd emphasize many of the same thoughts I shared with Jimmy above, but I'd also say this:

Amber, I'm sorry to tell you that you have a sexually transmitted infection. We're going to treat that aggressively. Meanwhile, what's done is done. You can't back up on the freeway of life, but I'm here to let you know that God wants you to be holy today. Each of us must live in holiness before the Lord in his or her own body. As the Bible teaches in Romans 14:12–13, "So then, each of us will give an account of himself to God. Therefore let us stop passing judgment on one another. Instead, make up your mind not to put any stumbling block or obstacle in your brother's way." Another important Bible verse says it well. Proverbs 24:16 says, "Though a righteous man falls seven times, he rises again." You can get up off the floor as well.

You can commit yourself to God to remain pure until your wedding day and become a secondary virgin. If you repent, tell the Lord you're truly sorry, and take steps to avoid sexual behavior, you can become a virgin in the sight of God again. Once you confess your sin and ask for God's forgiveness, he'll forgive you and cleanse you from all unrighteousness—it's as though you've never had sex before from a spiritual perspective. There are still physical, emotional, and relational scars that may always be there, but nevertheless, the Lord tells us in Isaiah 43:25, "I, even I, am he who blots out your transgressions, for my own sake, and remembers your sins no more."

That's a great promise you can take to the bank.

THE *M* WORD

I hope these sample talks were helpful to you. Now let's take a few pages to reflect on the sensitive topic of masturbation. You may have wondered if you should say anything to your teen about masturbation. You may be thinking that if you bring up the subject, you'll plant some ideas in your teen's head about trying out the practice. I'd advise you to broach the topic by the time your child turns twelve or thirteen. After that, the hormones really crank up, and they've probably heard plenty of stories from their friends, so if they don't hear something from you, they may be getting some inaccurate information.

First of all, I want to consider masturbation from a medical perspective. I have found no scientific evidence to indicate that this act is harmful to the body. It does not cause blindness, mental retardation, or warts to grow on the hand. These are old wives' tales. However, there can be emotional and spiritual effects. Masturbation sometimes causes oppressive guilt from which a teen can't escape. This guilt has the potential to do considerable psychological and spiritual damage. It also can become extremely obsessive—it is repeated over and over and becomes uncontrollable, consuming a person's life.

There are a variety of opinions about masturbation among the few Christian writers who have addressed the issue. Their viewpoints run the gamut: some call masturbation a sexual sin, while others claim it's a gift from God.

Those who consider masturbation to be sinful generally point to the fact that it's a solo act. The premise is that God's intended purpose for sex is to join two people together in marriage. To these writers, masturbating would violate this purpose. Others opposed to masturbation believe that the practice facilitates lust and fantasy and creates an increase in sexual tension—coming down in the end to "the more you have, the more you want." Most Christians who believe masturbation is a sin quote what the Bible says about purity and lust. And they make an excellent point. After all, masturbation is usually accompanied by sexual fantasies or the use of pornography. I don't think there's necessarily anything wrong with thinking about sex, but I do think the Bible indicates a person's sexual imagination has to be controlled. Most people who masturbate harbor fantasies that are plainly immoral, and these should have no place in a Christian's life.

Other Christian authors and experts consider masturbation allowable. These experts support the premise that masturbation is part of human sexual development. They contend that, while masturbation is normally a solo act, it can nevertheless serve a preparatory function for sexual intercourse within marriage. These writers also suggest that, rather than increasing sexual tension, masturbation serves to lower sexual tension by allowing the release of pent-up sexual urges. The practice is seen as having a particularly useful place in helping young men who wish to manage their sexual drive while remaining celibate. Personally, I find this view less persuasive.

Even though Christian authors vary on their opinions about masturbation, they agree that Scripture is silent on the issue. Yet, the Bible isn't afraid to mention all sorts of other sexual situations—homosexuality, adultery, prostitution, rape, incest, sex with animals, and so forth. The fact is, there is no place in Scripture where masturbation is even mentioned, much less forbidden. This strikes me as odd, since it's is a common human experience and the Bible does speak of other sexual sins (some fairly perverse and rare) without any reticence at all.

The book *Every Young Man's Battle* has an excellent viewpoint worth considering. Coauthors Steve Arterburn and Fred Stoeker make this observation:

> Since God didn't address masturbation directly in Scripture, the questions can seem endless. Theologians will argue over this until Christ returns, and maybe that's how it should be whenever Scripture is silent. Even we as coauthors have found it difficult to decide together what to label masturbation and where to draw the lines of sin.
>
> I (Fred) feel most comfortable simply calling masturbation a "sin" because its effects are exactly like the effects of any other sin in a man's life. If it looks like a duck, walks like a duck, and quacks like a duck, it likely *is* a duck:
>
> ❖ Habitual masturbation consistently creates distance from God.
> ❖ Jesus said that lusting after women in your heart is the same as doing it. Since most masturbation involves a lustful fantasy or pornography, we're certain that nearly all instances violate Scripture.
> ❖ Habitual masturbation is hard to stop. If you don't believe it, wait until you get married and try to quit masturbating.
> ❖ Masturbation is progressive. You're more likely to masturbate the day after you masturbate than you're likely to do it the day after you didn't.

Arterburn and Stoeker recommend four things young people should do:

1. Make a strong decision to not stop short of God's standards.
2. Join an accountability group that allows for the honest expression of feelings.

3. Continue an active ongoing relationship with God that involves worship and prayer.
4. Become aware of how various media—magazines, cable TV, videos, Internet, and sexy catalogs—affect your sex drive.

According to Arterburn and Stoeker, fulfilling these four requirements will allow you to love God with all your heart and strength. They conclude that at the end of the day, there are two questions that matter: If you're in bondage to masturbation, should you try to break free? Absolutely. Is it possible to break free? They believe it is, and it begins with a commitment not to masturbate today.

I'll give the last word on this discussion to Dr. James Dobson:

> What should you as a father say to your thirteen-year-old son about this subject? My advice is to say nothing after puberty has occurred. You will only cause embarrassment and discomfort. For those who are younger, it would be wise to include the subject of masturbation in the "Preparing for Adolescence" conversation I have recommended on other occasions. I would suggest that parents talk to their twelve- or thirteen-year-old boys, especially, in the same general way my mother and father discussed this subject with me.
>
> We were riding in the car, and my dad said, "Jim, when I was a boy, I worried so much about masturbation. It really became a scary thing for me because I thought God was condemning me for what I couldn't help. So I'm telling you now that I hope you don't feel the need to engage in this act when you reach the teen years, but if you do, you shouldn't be too concerned about it. I don't believe it has much to do with your relationship with God."
>
> What a compassionate thing my father did for me that night in the car. He was a very conservative minister who never compromised his standards of morality to the day of his death. He stood like a rock for biblical principles and commandments. Yet he cared enough about me to lift from my shoulders the burden of guilt that nearly destroyed some of my friends in the church. This kind of "reasonable" faith taught to me by my parents is one of the primary reasons I never felt it necessary to rebel against parental authority or defy God.
>
> Those are my views, for what they are worth. I know my recommendations will be inflammatory to some people. If you are one of them, please forgive me. I can only offer the best advice of which I'm capable. I pray that in this instance I am right.

ABOUT HOMOSEXUALITY

Let's keep marching on now and discuss the issue of homosexuality. When I was growing up in the Deep South, homosexuality was known as the "love that dare not speaketh its name." Now it's out there, front and center, in our culture, and gays and lesbians coming out of the closet these days receive a collective shrug. Homosexuals, who began making a push for tolerance twenty years ago, are now asking for acceptance and for the right to marry. People on both sides of the issue agree that we're in the midst of a culture war on this topic.

So parents, some teens will be drawn to what they perceive to be the glamour and excitement of an alternative lifestyle. Others will wonder if they are gay. A vast majority of teens—probably 98 percent, from the research I've seen—are heterosexuals and will be the rest of their lives.

Some concerned parents wonder about the position statements of major mental health organizations that claim there is no scientific evidence that a homosexual orientation can be changed by psychotherapy—often referred to as "reparative therapy." I do not believe there is good evidence to accept these statements.

Robert Spitzer, M.D., the psychiatrist known as the architect of the 1973 diagnostic manual that normalized homosexuality, recently expressed serious concern about the movement against sexual reorientation therapy. He cites findings from his own research: "I'm convinced from people I have interviewed ... many of them ... have made substantial changes toward becoming heterosexual. I came to this study skeptical. I now claim that these changes can be sustained."

What changed Dr. Spitzer's mind? He conducted a very elaborate study of 143 males and 57 females who had reported at least some minimal change from homosexual to heterosexual orientation that lasted at least five years. The majority of participants gave reports of change from a predominantly or exclusively homosexual orientation before therapy to a predominantly or exclusively heterosexual orientation in the year after the study. "There is evidence that change in sexual orientation following some form of reparative therapy does occur in some gay men and lesbians," he concluded.

At this point it would be instructive to bring Dr. Joseph Nicolosi into the discussion. Dr. Nicolosi is the president of the National Association for Research and Therapy of Homosexuality (NARTH), a professional organization dedicated to researching and treating homosexuality. As a licensed psychologist, Dr. Nicolosi has treated a wide variety of clients and specializes in treating homosexual men who are dissatisfied with their orientation and now believe treatment to change homosexuality can be effective and valuable.

I met Dr. Nicolosi when he was in Colorado Springs for the filming of Dr. James Dobson's "Bringing Up Boys" video series. Dr. Nicolosi was asked to share findings and information from his book *A Parent's Guide to Preventing Homosexuality*, which explains the critical role of fathers in raising boys with a healthy sexual identity. He says that when a boy sees his male role model—his father—as both good and strong, and the two of them share a masculine identity, gender confusion becomes less likely. It's also important for a father to have a warm relationship with his daughter because a dad can affirm his daughter's femininity.

Dr. Nicolosi allowed me to share his helpful answers to a few questions about homosexuality.

Q. Is homosexuality a choice?

A. Sexual inclinations and desires are never a "choice." Homosexuality originates from unconscious psychodynamic conflicts and many other early influences, including later habituation. But the individual does have a degree of choice in how he responds to his feelings and attractions.

Q. If a student has homosexual thoughts, feelings, or fantasies, does that mean he or she is gay or lesbian?

A. The teen years serve as a transitional phase when affectional, emotional, and identification needs can easily be eroticized.

Many factors can lead a questioning youngster into homosexual behavior, including curiosity, loneliness, need for attention, and desire for a sense of belonging. Gender-nonconforming boys often idealize other boys due to a sense of masculine inadequacy. Some girls are seeking the feminine nurturing and support they did not get from their mothers. Other boys retreat into the gay community where impersonal sex is readily available because of fear of the challenging social structure of heterosexual society. Still others were molested as children and are convinced they must be gay to have attracted a same-sex molester.

Q. Is there a "gay gene," and are people simply born gay?

A. Most gay-affirming programs promote this idea that homosexuality is inborn and unchangeable. This claim is based on some studies, which suggest that there may be a genetic predisposition to homosexuality.

However, no research has proven a person to be predetermined to be homosexual. Psychiatrist Jeffrey Satinover says, "There is no evidence that shows that homosexuality is genetic—and none of the research itself claims there is. Only the press and certain researchers do, when speaking in sound bites to the public.

"Like all complex behavioral and mental states, homosexuality is ... neither exclusively biological nor exclusively psychological, but results from a ... mixture of genetic factors, intrauterine influences, ... postnatal environment (such as parent, sibling and cultural behavior) and a complex series of repeatedly reinforced choices occurring at critical phases of development."

Is Dr. Nicolosi alone in his "politically incorrect" assessments about the roots and treatment of homosexuality? He is not. The Christian Medical Association has developed a comprehensive statement on homosexuality, which you can find (along with its extensive documentation) at www.highlyhealthy.net.

Here are a few of their medical and social conclusions about this controversial issue:

❖ The causes of same-sex attraction appear to be multi-factorial and may include developmental, psychosocial, environmental, and biological factors. There is no credible evidence at this time that same-sex attraction is genetically determined.

❖ Homosexual behavior can be changed. There is valid evidence that many individuals who desired to abstain from homosexual acts have been able to do so.

❖ Some homosexual acts are physically harmful because they disregard normal human anatomy and function. These acts are associated with increased risks of tissue injury, organ malfunction, and infectious diseases. These and other factors result in a significantly shortened life expectancy.

❖ Homosexual relationships are typically brief in duration. Homosexual behavior is destructive to the structures necessary for healthy marriages, families, and society. Men who commit homosexual acts have a high incidence of promiscuity, child molestation, and sexually transmitted infections. Homosexual behaviors burden society with increased medical costs, increased disability, and loss of productivity.

❖ Legalizing or blessing same-sex marriage or civil unions is harmful to the stability of society, the raising of children and the institution of marriage. If the only criterion for marriage were mutual consent or commitment, there are no grounds to prohibit polygamy, polyandry, or incestuous unions.

The Christian Medical Association draws these conclusions:

- ❖ The Christian community must respond to the complex issues surrounding homosexuality with grace, civility, and love.
- ❖ Christian doctors in particular must care for their patients involved in homosexual behavior in a nondiscriminating and compassionate manner, consistent with biblical principles.
- ❖ Anyone struggling with homosexual temptation should evoke neither scorn nor enmity, but evoke our concern, compassion, help, and understanding.
- ❖ The Christian community must condemn hatred and violence directed against those involved in homosexual behavior.
- ❖ The Christian community should oppose the legalization of same-sex marriage and/or blessing and adoption into homosexual environments.
- ❖ God provides the remedy for all moral failure through faith in Jesus Christ and the life-changing power of the Holy Spirit.

These observations and conclusions may not be popular, but they are medically reliable and biblically sound—a rarity in today's politically charged debate about homosexuality. I just thought you'd want the facts—fair and balanced.

Phew! We covered some heavy topics in this chapter, but it's the reality we face in the real world. Please remember that if you, the parent, don't speak up during the teachable moments, the world's megaphone is all they will hear. Perhaps having your teen read this section will be a good way to get the discussion ball rolling.

Well, we're getting there. Teens will need their spiritual wheels nice and full when it comes to the pressures they face in life. In the next chapter, I'll talk about the desperate need of teens to have a God-centered foundation on which to build as they continue their journey.

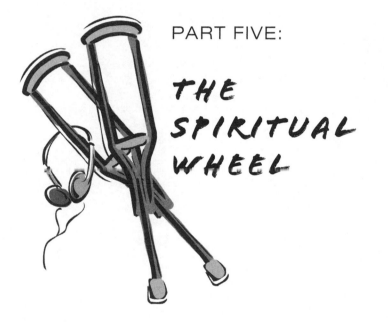

PART FIVE:

THE
SPIRITUAL
WHEEL

Chapter 14

BUILDING ON THE SOLID ROCK

I've long believed a healthy spiritual foundation is an essential component of highly healthy teens. It's visible in self-confident, highly healthy teens who know who they are and where they are going. This healthy spiritual foundation comes from knowing they are created and loved by God, with whom they have a personal relationship. Their parents have taught them that their Creator has endowed them with unique gifts, talents, and abilities. This foundation, which influences every part of a teen's life, is a magnificent resource a young person can draw on for a lifetime.

Like their parents, teens need a personal connection with God. They will benefit from understanding what the Bible says about them and how God's love for them is unconditional. Discovering and developing their spiritual gifts will help them live life to the fullest. Those who enter the young adult years without spiritual moorings, however, often drift through rocky waters during their twenties. A leaky personal relationship with God may shipwreck their boat before they reach the safe harbor of adulthood. Teens desperately need a healthy, God-centered foundation and outlook; otherwise, they could enter the adult years still trying to figure out life and their place in it. They need to hear from their parents how special they are to the Creator, who has a special plan for their lives.

I can't overemphasize how important it is for your teen's spiritual wheel to be filled with plenty of air during his or her adolescent years. If his or her tire is running low in this area, it can become quite difficult to pump it up with spiritual values *after* your teen leaves home. I don't want to say it's now or never for Christian parents, but according to an International Bible Society survey, 83 percent of all Christians make their personal commitment to God between the ages of four and fourteen. The Barna Group conducted a survey demonstrating that American children ages five to thirteen have a 32 percent probability of accepting Christ, but only a 6 percent chance when they're adults. Other studies indicate that the overwhelming majority of those who accept Christ do so before the age of eighteen.

I can't think of anything more important than leading your children into a personal relationship with Christ before they leave home. My collaborative writer Mike Yorkey coauthored a book titled *Faithful Parents, Faithful Kids*, in which they surveyed hundreds of adult children and asked them how their parents raised them. They heard stories of kids who rejected their parents' faith, no matter how much spiritual input was given, and they heard heartwarming stories of things parents did right.

Those who said they made it into their adult years with their faith intact rattled off dozens of ways their parents pointed them to a personal relationship with God. I'm going to list the top ten. (See if you can guess which response was number 1.)

1. We often heard conversational prayer in our home.
2. I always saw Mom and Dad reading their Bibles.
3. My parents taught us how to have a quiet time with the Lord each day.
4. We had easy access to Christian books and magazines.
5. Going to church on Sunday was a must.
6. We always had family devotions.
7. I made a profession of faith early in life.
8. What really helped was belonging to a great youth group during the teen years.
9. Every summer, I went to a Christian sports camp.
10. Other adults had a direct influence in pointing me toward Christ.

And the most popular response was—the envelope please—number 10! More than 90 percent of young adults surveyed said significant adults in their lives influenced them toward a relationship with God—Sunday school teachers, youth group leaders, Christian artists, aunts, uncles, brothers, sisters, grandparents, schoolteachers, and friends of the family.

Does this mean, then, that parents are only supporting cast members in leading their children to Christ? Not at all, especially because another Barna Research survey found that 47 percent of teens said their parents had their greatest influence on their spiritual development. What Johnson and Yorkey are saying is teens may hear from you and see a Christian life modeled in you, but when it comes to securing their commitment to God in their hearts and minds, they may feel more comfortable going forward, if you will, in the company of other family members or other significant people in their lives.

This was the case for Barb and me. We both grew up in homes that valued Sunday morning worship. We both attended Sunday school and church camps, but neither of us made a personal commitment to God until we were in college—a relationship that changed our lives forever. Nevertheless, we can look back now and see how valuable a relationship with God would have been in our childhood and teen years. Consequently, we wanted not only to model spiritual disciplines but also to encourage our children to make a commitment to a personal relationship with God early in their lives.

Barb and I shared our faith with Kate and Scott continuously. We prayed as a family. We worshiped as a family. We attended church picnics and fellowships as a family. We read Bible stories to our kids and prayed with them before meals and at bedtimes. We shared with them how we came to know God and the transforming impact he had on our lives and in our marriage. We reviewed spiritual principles and applied them to our family.

From time to time we taught our children the basic elements of the gospel: that God had a plan for their lives, but their (and all of our) wrongdoing caused them to become separated from God and unable to know him personally. However, God loved us enough to send his only Son, Jesus, to model a perfect life on earth and then to die a horrible death on our behalf—to pay the penalty for our sins and to pave the way for us to have a personal relationship with God and to enjoy eternal life with him in heaven.

We taught our kids that this relationship began when they chose to trust God with their lives, their decisions, and their futures—when they would recognize and admit that they (like their parents) were sinners in need of a Savior. We told them that when they were ready to make this commitment, we'd be there for them.

Kate's decision came when she was around five years old. One afternoon, while she and Barb were talking about God's plan for her life, Kate said she wanted to pray and ask Jesus to come into her heart. She and her mom prayed together, and then Barb and Kate came over to my medical office to let me know what had happened. Scott's decision, also at about age five, came one evening when he and I were watching Kate taking part in a gymnastics exercise. We were talking about a Bible story at the time, and he looked up at me and said, "Dad, I want to have Jesus in my heart." We talked about it a bit more, and then we prayed together at the side of the gym.

Barb and I took seriously the Bible's instruction that we were to teach them biblical principles and lessons at all times. In the Old Testament book of Deuteronomy, this is what God's Word says:

> *Hear, O Israel: The LORD our God, the LORD is one. Love the LORD your God with all your heart and with all your soul and with all your strength. These commandments that I give you today are to be upon your hearts. Impress them on your children. Talk about them when you sit at home and when you walk along the road, when you lie down and when you get up. Tie them as symbols on your hands and bind them on your foreheads. Write them on the doorframes of your houses and on your gates.*
>
> *Deuteronomy 6:4–9*

We believed this biblical instruction was not for rabbis, pastors, or priests but for parents.

It's tempting for parents of teens to let others—pastors, youth pastors, Sunday school teachers—give our children their spiritual training. Many parents believe that if they take their teens to a church to receive spiritual training from a pastoral professional or committed layperson, their adolescents will turn out all right. It can happen, but it's not nearly as life changing or effective as when parents take charge of this God-given responsibility.

Pastoral professionals may have more knowledge of spiritual things than a typical mom or dad, but they don't (and aren't supposed to) have the heart attachment that parents have for their children. The average pastoral professional will never have the quality and quantity of time parents should have with their children. A faith community can supplement the spiritual foundation laid at home, but it can never replace it!

As our children were growing up, we tried to love them unconditionally and to create the atmosphere in which they could make their decision about the gospel. Let me be clear about this: the decision was *theirs*, not ours. Choosing to have a personal relationship with God through Christ in no way resulted in any rewards or privileges. We didn't want to coerce our children into a counterfeit relationship. Instead, we wanted to pray for and encourage them—when *they* were ready—to know God the way we did.

TEENS' PURPOSE IN LIFE

During my two decades of medical practice, I observed that some teens were well on the road toward living life with a simple creed: "I am born; I live; I die." Their fatalism was nurtured in a culture that pays homage to how much stuff can be accumulated and how many pleasurable things can be crammed into a weekend. It's an empty way to go through life, and when the dust settles, young adults are sure to experience disillusionment and sadness. The bottom line for many teens is this: they don't realize they need a spiritual foundation to mitigate these feelings of emptiness.

Without some sort of spiritual anchor, teens bob like a cork in a polluted cultural ocean that has become increasingly hostile to religious beliefs. Many leaders of our cultural institutions no longer encourage and support spiritual health. Many in the world of academia, who have pinned their hopes on Darwinian evolution, often deny the existence of a Creator. Hollywood is rarely friendly to characters with Christian values. Our nation's judges, misinterpreting the freedom of religion in our Bill of Rights, have virtually banned religious expression from the public square. Some students are told they don't have the right to bow their heads and say a prayer in the school cafeteria, carry a Bible on campus, or participate in student-led religious groups on school grounds.

FYI . . .   ⏪ ▶ ⏸ ⏹ ⏩

► Psychologist Andrew Weaver studied the way religious or spiritual experience affects a teen's behavior and development. He concluded that a teen's spiritual foundation serves as a buffer from the cultural and social poisons of modern life. He found that religious belief among teens portends many healthy outcomes, including reduced suicide, less depression, better response to trauma, reduced nonmarital sex and pregnancy, and less substance abuse. What's more, religious faith can give teens a sense of hope and a higher purpose in life.

True Spirituality

I'm not prepared, however, to say that the sky is falling. After the Columbine High and September 11 tragedies, students flocked to religious leaders and religious institutions seeking comfort. These teens wanted more than a pat on the shoulder; they wanted someone to tell them about the hope they can have in God and about true spirituality.

In fact, national surveys show that the natural tendency of teens is to be religious. Here are just a few facts from the Barna Group:

- ❖ Nearly nine out of ten (89 percent) teens pray weekly.
- ❖ Over half of teens (56 percent) attend church on a given Sunday.
- ❖ 38 percent of teens donate some of their own money to a church in a given week.
- ❖ 35 percent of teens attend Sunday school in a given week.
- ❖ 35 percent of teens read the Bible each week, not including when they are in church.
- ❖ More than seven out of ten teens are engaged in some church-related effort in a typical week: attending worship services, Sunday school, a church youth group, or a small group.
- ❖ 32 percent of teens attend youth group, other than a small group or Sunday school, each week.

My guess is that the difference in these high rates of religious activity in teens and much lower rates in adults is due to one of two reasons: (1) More teens are finding a personal relationship with God than their parents did, or (2) Many of these teens are involved in religion without having a personal relationship with God—in other words, they're looking for something that is deeply satisfying and not finding it in religious activity. Let me explain.

The concept of true spirituality is clearly outlined in the Bible. God's Word says that true spirituality involves an authentic, growing personal relationship with a personal God. It doesn't matter what race, ethnicity, economic status, or class you are because spirituality promotes the wellness and welfare of everyone. True spirituality is the sum of one's beliefs and values that can be seen in the way we display the spiritual fruit of love, joy, peace, patience, kindness, goodness, faithfulness, gentleness, and self-control.

These are great attributes for every teen, and research shows that highly healthy adolescents who have a foundation of true spirituality frequently pray, apply the Bible's truths to daily life, believe they have a personal relationship with God, and are more apt to practice what they preach.

Not all spiritual foundations are equal, however. Consider these differences among those who say they are part of a faith community:

❖ Some religions separate people from their families and their communities or encourage blind devotion and obedience to a single charismatic leader—think of Jim Jones forcing his flock to drink poisoned Kool-Aid in Jonestown, Guyana.

❖ Christmas and Easter church attendees—those who go through the motions of religious tradition—tend to experience an external faith that is less likely to be associated with positive health outcomes. The benefits of true spirituality are generally lost on them because they are using religion to serve themselves, not to serve God.

❖ Religion that fosters true spirituality is likely to be highly healthy, in contrast to religion that is negative or done for show. This helps explain why true spirituality is such a powerful force in regulating behavior. Those who take their spirituality to heart live out a moral value system that results in positive or healthy outward behavior.

Cassie's Story

A teen named Cassie Bernall is a great example of how true spirituality became the anchor she needed in a life-or-death moment. Cassie may have been just another Columbine High student on the morning of April 20, 1999, but she had something extra in her heart after she accepted Christ two years before that fateful day. Whereas she had been a troubled teen dabbling in witchcraft and isolating herself from others, Cassie's newfound faith took her in a much more positive direction. She knew who she was—a child of God.

I can't imagine the horror of that morning, of gunshots echoing in the air, followed by anguished screams and pleas for help. Eyewitnesses tell us that Eric Harris and Dylan Klebold caught up with Cassie, and one of them had a question for her—a question that would determine whether or not she lived.

"Do you believe in God?" one of the killers asked.

Cassie never hesitated. "Yes," she replied.

"Why?" she was asked, but before she could answer, she was shot in the head.

Cassie's dramatic story underscores the power of a spiritual foundation to help anchor a teen's life and turn it around from being highly unhealthy to becoming highly healthy. Her killers, on the other hand, had deeply immersed themselves in a different kind of spirituality. They embraced the dark elements of Nazism and the nihilism of Nietzsche, and they consumed a steady diet of death-themed music, film, and video games. They reaped what they had sown in their hearts.

I think it's impossible for teens to become highly healthy without a foundation of positive spirituality in their lives—and I'm convinced it can only happen when teens choose to begin a personal relationship with God (or to deepen that relationship during the teen years if it began in childhood). When teens adopt true spirituality, it helps them resist doing self-destructive things and brings them closer to God, and it's more likely to result in a life that manifests joy, peace, and satisfaction. Furthermore, they'll be much better off because a spiritual foundation is associated with improved physical, emotional, and relational health. Knowing that God loves them can help reduce stress, and reduced stress can result in less anxiety and teen depression.

THE POWER OF A YOUTH GROUP

One of the best ways to build a spiritual foundation is to get your teens involved in a great youth group. Barb and I wanted Kate and Scott to choose a group that would share our attitudes about believing in Jesus Christ as Lord and Savior, understand the role of the Holy Spirit's work in their lives, and love and obey God. Just as we did, you're undoubtedly hoping that your teen finds his or her purpose in life—the answer to that all-encompassing question "What on earth am I here for?"

This is a profound question, and I realize many parents may still be trying to figure out the answer for themselves. There is a famous story about the great poet Lord Byron writing in his diary, "I go to bed with a heaviness of heart at having lived so long with so little purpose." We all come from different spiritual backgrounds and have different levels of spiritual maturity. Some of you may be veteran Christians. Others may have just become followers of Jesus Christ. You may be playing catch-up and looking for ways to make sure your teens' spiritual wheels are staying well inflated. The wonderful thing is that the Lord has promised to meet us right where we are. It doesn't matter how spiritually mature or how spiritually inexperienced you are. God has promised to work with us, and when he's working in your life, you can be sure he's working in your teens' lives as well.

There's no doubt that the teen years are easier on everyone when both parents and teens are riding on well-inflated spiritual wheels. But even then, we'll still run into some potholes along the way because that's part of life. Simply put, if you or your teens aren't currently in the midst of some storm or crisis, you can be sure one's coming somewhere down the pike!

FAITH DEVELOPMENT

The adolescent years are years of discovering new things and of asking questions. Even if your children have been going to church since infancy and starred as the baby Jesus or Joseph in the Christmas pageant (or the Virgin Mary, as Kate did), there will be a crossroad in their teen years, if not earlier, when they'll have to decide either Jesus Christ is who he said he is—the Son of God who died on a cross to pay the penalty for their sins—or he isn't. As young people question the world around them, they no longer accept things at face value, nor do they believe in something just because we told them to. They must come to a point where they personally receive the gospel and accept Jesus Christ as their Savior based on the truths of the Bible.

Researchers have found common stages young people go through in their faith development. Jay Kesler, president emeritus of Taylor University, outlined four of these stages in his book *Energizing Your Teenager's Faith*:

- ❖ Children in grade school who talk about God are echoing the words they've heard from their parents and other adults in their lives. Important patterns of spiritual development are formed during these years.
- ❖ Junior highers have an *affiliated faith* that sees their beliefs in terms of a relationship. For instance, Jesus is their "best friend." Their faith grows mainly through church and youth group interaction.
- ❖ High schoolers develop a *searching faith*. Tough questions are asked to help them sort out whether to personally accept what they've experienced. This is the time when parents need to spend hours discussing these questions.
- ❖ Young adults begin to develop an *owned faith*. When they accept their Christian beliefs, these young adults adopt these biblical values as their own.

Barb and I recognized that Kate and Scott needed to take ownership of their faith in Christ sometime during their teen years. I described earlier how Kate and I would get up at 5:30 a.m. and have a quiet time of reading the Bible and praying together. When Kate started high school, Barb and I felt it was best for her to have her own prayer and quiet time. During this time of life, she discovered journaling. We'd buy the journals, and she'd chronicle her daily life and her relationship with God. It's still an important discipline for her today.

We encouraged Scott to interact with people we thought could be spiritual mentors and role models. It's interesting how your teens listen better to your friends who are saying exactly the same things you'd say—but because it's coming from someone other than good ol' Mom and Dad, they accept it as gospel truth. So every summer during Scott's junior high and high school days we were pleased to send him to Kamp Kanakuk, a Christian sports camp, where he was discipled by great speakers and caring counselors in his cabin. (I tip my hat to my good friends Joe and Debbie-Jo White, who oversee twelve Kanakuk camps hosting 20,000 campers and 2,500 college-age and professional staff members every summer—thereby influencing the next generation in a profound way.)

Combating Moral Relativism

One of Kamp Kanakuk's greatest strengths is its emphasis on absolute truth and a biblical worldview. Barb and I were pleased that God's absolute truth was reinforced at Kanakuk, because we were reminding our teens constantly that absolute standards of right and wrong could be found in the truth of God's Word.

This has been a controversial concept since the 1960s—when *Time* magazine's cover asked, "Is God Dead?" It became popular to believe that no one can have a monopoly on truth as it relates to values or ethics, because who can say their truth is better than someone else's truth? This led to the current prevailing philosophy that everything is dependent on one's feelings and belief system at that particular moment, and thus there's no such thing as truth or certainty in our lives.

Moral relativism says that what may be right for you may not be right for me, that what may be wrong for you may not be wrong for me. We all coexist with our own versions of the truth because truth is what *feels* right to the individual. From a young age, I learned that Jesus Christ is the same "yesterday and today and forever," as the Bible tells us in Hebrews 13:8. As Kate and Scott became teens, I pointed out that God's Word *has* to be our ultimate source for what's absolutely true about God—for what we believe in and stake our lives on.

When I talk before a group of teens, I like to share this illustration. I tell them to imagine camping on a river. We are two miles below a very large dam. The camp ranger has just received a radio message that the dam has broken. In exactly two minutes, he says, the valley will be flooded by a rushing and raging torrent of water. To save ourselves, we're told, we have to run due north up the side of the valley. It's the only way we can escape the surging water and live.

Then I have the teens close their eyes and put one hand over their eyes. "With your other hand, I want you to point north," I say. "May I remind you that your life depends on getting this right. If you're off just a little bit, you'll die. Everyone pointing north? Good. Now please open your eyes."

The kids almost always giggle because invariably they're all pointing in different directions.

"Ladies and gentlemen, there's only one true north, and we're going to find out what it is. Please keep pointing in the direction you think is north while I pull out this trusty compass."

I gaze at my compass and say, "North is thataway!" The kids laugh again because so few got it right. When the room settles down, I say, "Everyone who is pointing due north, I want you to stand up."

Typically only a handful of geographically minded teens stand, and when they do, I say, "You live! The rest of you, I want you to lie down and cross your arms over your chests because you are *dead!*"

The point is clear: there is such a thing as absolute truth. Go true north, and you escape the rampaging waters. Go in another direction, and you're flotsam. Yet most teens don't see life this way. In a 2001 survey conducted by the Barna Group, 83 percent of teens maintain that moral truth depends on the circumstances, and only 6 percent believe moral truth is absolute. For those teens who said they were Christians (and Barna asked certain questions to determine how real their faith was to them), their responses were better but not by much: 9 percent of the teens said moral truth doesn't change, a substantial number (76 percent) said moral truth depends on the situation, and 15 percent said they didn't know. Only 9 percent of Christian teens get it when it comes to absolute truth? And 15 percent of Christian kids say they don't know one way or another? This is not good news.

It's cut-and-dried for me: Jesus is truth. He declared in John 14:6, "I am the way and the truth and the life. No one comes to the Father except through me." In John 8:31–32, Jesus said to those Jews who had believed in him, "If you hold to my teaching, you are really my disciples. Then you will know the truth, and the truth will set you free."

Here's another story that communicates effectively to teens. Imagine you're standing on the edge of an alpine lake. The frigid water is covered with ice. You believe with all your heart—you *totally* believe—that the ice will hold you up. When you step out on it, however, it's only one-sixteenth of an inch thick. Guess what? No matter how strong your belief, you're going to get very cold and very wet. Now suppose your belief is very weak and shallow, but the ice is three feet thick. Guess what? You'll be enjoying smooth and dry skating. Here's the upshot: the object in which you place your faith is more important than the degree of faith you have. Thus, I'm placing my faith in the absolute truth.

If you and your teens are rooted in God's Word and the spiritual disciplines, you will find truth, your lives will be anchored, and you will bear fruit. Guaranteed.

PLUGGED IN

When Kate and Scott entered the teen years, their taste in music changed as fast as they outgrew their old Nikes. No longer were simple Christian ditties or childhood songs interesting to them. They wanted fast-paced music with a beat—especially Scott.

As Christian parents we cared a lot about both the media images our children saw and the music they listened to. We didn't want Kate and Scott to develop a taste for Marilyn Manson, Tupac Shakur, Alanis Morissette, and other secular musicians popular in the latter half of the 1990s. We preferred they listen to great Christian music, even if it had a strong beat. You can find just about every genre of music—including that awful rap (did I say that?)—represented in Christian music. So if your teens have developed a taste for punk rock, you can find a Christian alternative that has positive, even worshipful lyrics.

To me, lyrics are the big deal; style of music isn't. Pastor Rick Warren, writing in *The Purpose-Driven Life*, says it's the words that make a song sacred, not the tune:

> Christians often disagree over the style of music used in worship, passionately defending their preferred style as the most biblical or God-honoring. But there is no biblical style! There are no musical notes in the Bible; we don't even have the musical instruments they used in Bible times.

Frankly, the music style you like best says more about *you*—your background and personality—than it does about God. One ethnic group's music can sound like noise to another. But God likes variety and enjoys it all.

You need to get plugged in, so look no further than Focus on the Family's Plugged In website (link to it from my website at www.highlyhealthy.net) to find out the great artists your teens would enjoy and the ones to avoid. Take the time to read the lyrics pages to determine if the words emphasize harmful actions or promote immediate gratification.

If you're late arriving to this party and your teens have towers of questionable CDs in their bedrooms, I'd advise you to swallow hard and offer to buy back their CDs, urging them to use the money to buy positive Christian alternatives. Sit down with your teen and read the lyrics written by these secular artists. Observe that rappers spewing the "*F* word" and "ho's" don't meet the family standard.

Music is a powerful medium, nearly as strong as movies. If you don't agree, then turn on an oldies station the next time you're in the car and listen to some of your old favorite songs. Notice how you remember all the words, even if it's been fifteen or twenty years since you last heard the song. Believe me, if you heard Rod Stewart's raspy voice on "Do Ya Think I'm Sexy?" you'll remember those words!

LISTEN UP!

Not only must we teach the truth to our teens, we must demonstrate the truth by example—truth taught as well as truth lived out. Barb and I enjoyed a nightly prayer time with our children from their earliest days and on through their teen years. This rich interaction had become a sweet time of listening to them talk about their day or about the things they were looking forward to. Even in their high school years, we hugged and kissed them as we tucked them in and ended the day with a prayer.

Dr. Walt Larimore

SPIRITUALLY ANCHORED

Barb and I always placed an extremely high value on worshiping God as a family. We felt if the choice came down to a church where our teens felt comfortable in their youth program versus a church we especially liked, we'd make the sacrifice for them. And that's just what happened. When Kate and Scott were in their teen years, we gravitated toward a church with one of the best youth groups in the county—good youth pastors, strong programs, great missions emphasis, and a robust discipleship program. We felt that the spiritual anchor was critical during those years, which reminds me of Hebrews 6:19—our hope in God is like "an anchor for the soul, firm and secure."

In the old sailing days on the Mediterranean Sea, most of the harbors were very small, especially on the islands where rocks jutted out of the water. Whenever a storm was in the air, these small harbors would quickly fill with boats—so many, sometimes, that they didn't have room for every boat that was seeking refuge from the coming storm. When too many boats had congregated, the harbormaster would send out a small boat—a forerunner or anchor runner—to meet the larger vessel. The forerunner would take the boat's anchor and drop it in the shallower and rockier harbor, thus giving the larger vessel a safe haven of sorts from the coming storm.

That's a great picture for parents of teens. The forerunner boat takes our anchor—which is the hope we have for our teens—and places it in the harbor, even though we can't see its exact location. We knew that our anchor was secure as long as it was remaining anchored spiritually and keeping our kids tied to us. No matter what the storm, that's the type of anchor we want. It gives us security, and it gives us hope.

Your efforts will have profound impact, I can assure you. This point was driven home to me a couple of years ago when Kate was working in Washington, D.C., as a White House intern. Barb, Scott, and I flew to our nation's capital at Thanksgiving time so we could spend time together and see where Kate hung out at 1600 Pennsylvania Avenue.

We were impressed, and Barb and I were so proud of her. We went out for Thanksgiving dinner that night and listened to Kate—and then Scott—tell story after story after story about growing up. You know how kids can get on a roll as they laugh and say, "Yeah, but you remember when . . ." It seemed as though they tried to top each other for more than an hour.

Later that evening at our hotel, Barb asked an interesting question: "Did you notice how many of their memories involved church or our family's spiritual activities?"

I thought for a moment and realized she was right. "Yes!" I exclaimed.

That evening, as we went to bed, Barb and I thanked the Lord that our children's spiritual wheels were full of air. I was reminded of the verse in the Bible that says, "For physical training [the physical wheel] is of some value, but godliness [the spiritual wheel] has value for all things, holding promise for both the present life and the life to come." Then we both fell asleep with big, satisfied grins on our faces.

Well, we're nearly done now. In the last chapter I'll talk about how to give your teens the skills they'll need when they leave home for college or for whatever big adventure God has waiting for them. Then you'll be ready for perhaps your most difficult assignment—letting go!

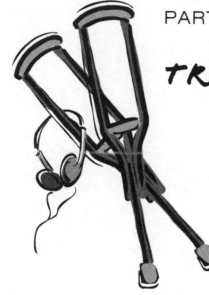

PART SIX:

TRANSITIONS

Chapter 15

INTO THE CLUBHOUSE TURN

I've delivered over 1,500 babies into the world, and each one was completely helpless the moment he or she drew the first breath. Those infants began life in a state of complete dependence, needing someone to feed them, change them, bathe them, and clothe them.

Eighteen years later, they are no longer helpless. They've become young adults, capable of feeding and clothing themselves and eager to experience what life holds for them. Some stay home and join the ranks of the employed, while others attend a trade school or a community college. Some leave the nest and enroll in college, where they experience independence for the first time. They—and only they—are responsible for signing up for classes, taking notes, doing homework, studying for tests, making sure they get enough of the right foods to eat, managing their money wisely, and keeping themselves highly healthy.

Every parent's goal should be to work himself or herself out of a job. We all understand we can't wait until the summer between high school graduation and freshman orientation week to teach our sons and daughters the importance of remaining sexually pure before marriage, staying away from drugs and alcohol, cultivating highly healthy friendships, developing a highly healthy lifestyle, and building a personal relationship with God. They need to be coached, coaxed, and cultured by us *throughout* their long flight of adolescence, not during the final approach.

WHEN THEY LEAVE HOME

At the outset of this book I noted that nurturing highly healthy teens is a process that takes you from being their health care quarterback to their health care coach. As your teens graduate from high school and move on to their first job or to the college dorms, it's your fervent hope that they'll leave home with all four wheels—physical, emotional, relational, and spiritual—fully inflated and well balanced for the ride ahead.

Ensuring Good Medical Care

At eighteen, the law states that our children are emancipated from their parents, but in medical terms, they've been free from parental control for several years in the area of sexual behavior. Minor children can obtain from many doctors pregnancy tests, birth control pills, birth control information, and treatment for STIs without your knowledge or permission. Nevertheless, as you set them free, your teens will be calling more of their own health care plays. If you've had a good relationship along the way and coached with encouragement, you'll still be involved.

I would recommend that your older teens retain the services of your family doctor until they are out of college and living on their own (perhaps in another community, if that's where God leads them to live). Your family doctor will have their history at his or her fingertips, as well as a mental note of the type of family care you expect. From an insurance standpoint, staying with your family doctor should be relatively simple, because most health care plans allow you to keep your college-age children on the family plan as long as they're full-time students.

FYI . . . ⏮ ▶ ⏸ ⏹ ⏭

▶ The U.S. Census Bureau reported in 2002 that young adults are the least likely to have health insurance. Nearly 30 percent of the eighteen- to twenty-four-year-olds nationwide are uninsured. It's easy to see how some young people get lost between the cracks. They lose parental coverage for one reason or another; perhaps they're looking for a good job that offers health insurance or they're finishing school. But more and more young people in their twenties are intentionally shunning health care coverage. They've been healthy all their lives, they say—and besides, medical coverage is too expensive and just for "old people."

Wrong on all counts. Yes, young people are healthy (that's why they pay the lowest rates), but they do get into accidents. Even a broken leg while snowboarding can cost between $5,000 and $10,000 in routine care. A car accident, God forbid, could set them back tens of thousands of dollars.

All things considered, health insurance for young adults is one of the better buys on the planet. Visit eHealthInsurance.com (you can access it at www.highlyhealthy.net), plug in your zip code, gender, and date of birth, and you'll see that decent health insurance can be had for under $50 a month. A twenty-four-year-old male living in my hometown of Monument, Colorado, in 2004, would pay $49.68 monthly for coverage with a $1,000 deductible and a co-insurance rate of 20 percent—but office visits wouldn't be covered. A female the same age would pay about $7 more per month. (Of course, one could pay a higher monthly rate and shell out less on the back end. That's the way it is for any health care plan.)

Bottom line: You don't want to go through life without health care insurance. An inopportune accident or illness can have a devastating impact on the short-term and long-term health of an individual. Even if an entry-level job doesn't include health care benefits, there's no excuse for not having coverage.

THE LONG BEGINNING

As I write this book, Kate and Scott are in their early- to mid-twenties. Because they're unmarried, Barb and I feel they remain under our care and protection to a certain extent. Sure, they're young adults, and like most parents, we're proud of who they've become and where they're going in life. We're convinced that God has a plan for their lives, and we're confident that his plan will eventually include marrying and forming their own families.

The Importance of Premarital Counseling

If and when Kate and Scott find that special person, our last parental act will be to urge the happy couple to go through extensive premarital counseling. In fact, Barb and I believe so strongly in premarital counseling that we'll spring for it—even if it costs $1,000. And I don't mean casual, drive-by premarital counseling, where two lovebirds slouch on the pastor's couch a week before the wedding and breeze through a premarital checklist. I'm talking about a full-blown premarital counseling experience, where couples explore the differences in their temperaments and discuss their expectations about everything from how many children they'd like to have to where they'll attend church. There are sexual adjustments to talk over, as well as their short-term and long-term career goals. Research is showing that couples who attend premarital counseling classes have lower divorce rates and score higher in marital satisfaction.

The Importance of a Premarital Physical Examination

My last word of advice for Kate and Scott before their wedding day would center around the importance of a premarital physical. Back in my parents' day, couples in many states were required to have a blood test before marriage, which screened for syphilis. While blood tests may have gone the way of rotary phones, I believe they still have great value.

I recommended prenuptial physicals in my practice whenever I heard a young adult was getting married. I stressed the importance of getting both bride and groom caught up in health maintenance and being sure all necessary screens were done and health care information updated. I considered it important for a woman to have her hymen checked to make sure the opening into the vagina was sufficiently unrestricted; otherwise, on her wedding night, her groom could tear the hymen during sexual intercourse, turning a pleasurable experience into a very painful one. (If young women use tampons in their teen years, however, they're far less likely to have a significant problem in this area.)

Whenever I did a premarital physical, I'd offer to meet with the couple to discuss their sexual relationship. The young couples were usually giddy with excitement because the big day was rapidly approaching, and I didn't want to do anything to temper that innocent joy. Nonetheless, there were realities to deal with, and one of the biggest was the first night in which they'd sleep together.

I encouraged a couple to wait a day or two after the wedding before leaving for the honeymoon. If they were getting married in the same town they were planning to live in, I strongly suggested they spend at least their first two nights in their apartment or home and not let anyone in the world know— except maybe one parent.

I was usually asked why. It was a great question, but I had a good reason for my advice. The wedding experience is so draining that to hustle from the reception to catch a flight or drive somewhere and then check into a hotel hours and hours later can be unnerving and exhausting. I'd look the guy in the eye and say, "Generally speaking, the way God designed a woman, her home is her nest. That's part of who she is and part of her security. So if your lovely wife-to-be has already decorated your apartment and personalized it for you, and you bring her home on her first night—to her nest—it can be an incredibly comfortable feeling for her." (If they were virgins, I added that having your first night together in your own bed would be especially memorable. Many couples later told me that no one had ever suggested this before, but they were glad they took me up on the advice.)

Most couples nod their heads, and then I drop the bomb. "The last thing I want to share is that you don't *have* to consummate your marriage on your wedding night." I usually receive a look of astonishment after making the statement, and then I turn my attention to the groom.

"Let me explain. There's a good chance your wife will be plum exhausted, so you don't have to force things. It's okay to hug and kiss and explore and fondle, but it's also okay to wait. If you don't have sex that night, that's fine. If you do, let her take control, even to the point that if she wants to be on top, let her. She can control the depth of penetration and the movement. Many times when a guy is on top, it's just so exciting, so thrilling, there's a chance he'll lose control and hurt her, which can be psychologically damaging. So my advice is, let her have control. Let her say yes, let her say no, and let her say when."

I also wanted the young couple to know that great sex is a learned activity. Many couples expect that the first experience will be perfect and totally satisfying. I let them know it seldom is—but that's okay. By lowering their expectations, sex can actually become more fun for them.

Let me share a suspicion with you: I rather doubt that any couples have taken my advice to wait until the next day to consummate their marriage. I'm fine with that. To me what's important is they heard the message that they didn't *have* to make love that night, and it took the pressure off. Learning that the first sexual experience didn't have to be perfect ratcheted down the pressure, making their first experience that much better.

CLOSING THOUGHTS

In the Bible, the psalmist wrote this about children:

Behold, children are a gift of the Lord,
The fruit of the womb is a reward.

Like arrows in the hand of a warrior,
So are the children of one's youth.
How blessed is the man whose quiver is full of them;
They will not be ashamed
When they speak with their enemies in the gate.

Years ago, during a morning quiet time, I was meditating on this great truth when it struck me that arrows were not designed to remain in the quiver; they were designed to be shot into the world. This concept got me thinking about my family and about the parents of the newborn babies, who needed to hear this message. Shortly after that, I began praying with parents in the delivery room after their newborn son or daughter had been born. With head bowed and eyes closed, I would say something like this:

Lord, thank you for the gift of this little baby—a person you designed and wove together in his mother's womb. I know this little one is of inestimable worth in your eyes. I pray for his mother and father, that they would be wise in raising him. I pray that they would assist him to come to know you and to make you known to others. I pray that he would love you with all his heart and soul and mind and strength and that he would love others as himself. Prepare his mom and dad, even now, for that day when they would launch him into the world. Give them the strength and wisdom to do just that. In Jesus' name. Amen.

I'll never forget the time Barb and I took Kate to college. She began her college career at Clearwater Christian College in Clearwater, Florida. Although we had a road trip ahead of us to get her there, we were *so* ready for that day. Barb and I felt no dread because we had been praying and preparing for eighteen years. That Friday morning, we packed up the minivan and hopped on the interstate. That afternoon, we arrived in Clearwater and spent the afternoon moving Kate into her apartment. We took her out to dinner and then back to her apartment, where we prayed together, and her mother and I blessed her. Our departing was tearful but joyful.

With the west coast of Florida in our rearview mirror, Barb and I were happy and pleased for Kate. We felt satisfaction that our work was done. After all, we had devoted ourselves for more than eighteen years, striving to be highly healthy parents who would raise highly healthy children and nurture highly healthy teens. As the mileage markers passed, I thought about how Barb and I were returning home to begin a new chapter in our lives, and it sounded exciting to me.

Then it happened—totally unexpected and a complete shock. Hot tears began rolling down my cheeks as I clenched the steering wheel. I struggled to concentrate as I drove at freeway speed. I thought of all our wonderful memories of raising Kate. My mind thumbed through a picture book of memories—her first steps, building sand castles at the beach, walking her to her first kindergarten class, receiving her prized "artwork" and taping it on the refrigerator door, and visiting the White House on a family trip to Washington, D.C. The memories prompted me to weep uncontrollably, and when Barb saw me crying, she unleashed a torrent of tears as well.

I pulled off the freeway and parked on the off-ramp shoulder. Barb and I leaned over and held each other close, sobbing in each other's arms. The reality that the childhood years were over hit us like a blow to the midsection.

Looking back, I know it was okay to cry—even therapeutic. When it's time to pack your oldest's belongings and help him or her move into the freshman dorm—or his or her first apartment—hopefully you'll have a lump in your throat as well. My hope is that when that special moment arrives, you won't look back with regret but with tears of happiness and poignancy, just as Barb and I did on that weekend—knowing that our teen had become a highly healthy adult. Her health wheels were inflated and balanced. She was ready to go.

I pray that your dearly loved child will be a healthy young adult, ready to be released into the arms of someone you know and trust—Jesus Christ.

Acknowledgments

I am grateful to the many people have contributed to this book. First and foremost, Mike Yorkey has been much more than my collaborative writer; he has become a special friend. He helped me craft a book that I hope any parent can not only enjoy reading but also use to effectively guide and nurture a highly healthy teen.

The staff at Zondervan, as always, has been both professional and encouraging. Cindy Lambert has been the shepherd for each book I've written. She has been a confidante, cheerleader, and critic. Her caring, coaching, and camaraderie have provided a valued gift. Her hand-holding and encouragement during every phase of this book's development were critical. Cindy is a magnificent editor and a very special friend.

Dirk Buursma, as usual, has pulled the final manuscript together beautifully. As a reader of this book, you will be the recipient of his commitment to high-quality editing. Sue Brower and her staff provide the marketing and public relations services that allow this book to get into the hands of as many parents as possible.

During my four years of practice in Bryson City, North Carolina, and my sixteen years in Kissimmee, Florida, my medical partners never ceased to teach me what it meant to be a doctor who inculcates highly healthy habits into the teens and parents for whom we cared. Rick Pyeritz, M.D., and John Hartman, M.D., were marvelous teachers, splendid partners, trusted confidants, and brilliant physicians. They were the family physicians for my children as they were growing up, and I'll forever appreciate their love and care for Kate and Scott. They are two of my dearest friends, and much of this book was cultivated while I was in practice with them.

During my years of medical practice, I was privileged to care for thousands of teens as they grew and developed. Many have now completed college and graduate school. Others have married and are beginning their families. The experience I gained, at their expense, benefits you because I learned many of these principles from them. I am so thankful to each of them. I have taken care to protect their privacy whenever I have shared their stories.

My executive assistant, Donna Lewis, unselfishly assisted in manuscript review and research arrangements. In addition, she organized many of the book's resource recommendations. Thanks, Donna, for your customary "above and beyond" work and dedication.

Rob Flanegin and Chris Baur envisioned and built the initial website for *God's Design for the Highly Healthy Person* (www.10essentials.net). Dr. Brad Beck, Barb Seibert, Char Carter, and Charlene Vernon all helped build and maintain the website for this book and also for *God's Design for the Highly Healthy Child* (www.highlyhealthy.net). Diane Passno and Ken Janzen at Focus on the Family spent hours reviewing the manuscript and making valuable suggestions.

Paul Batura helped with permissions and research. Drs. Gary Chapman and Joseph Nicolosi both kindly allowed me permission to use their words and concepts. I am indebted to the Christian Medical Association for their initiative in bringing the *Highly Healthy* books to print. David Stevens, M.D., and Gene Rudd, M.D., through their leadership roles and friendship, were actively involved in bringing this project to fruition.

Many thanks to those who took time to carefully review early drafts of the manuscript and offer suggestions that have improved the final product—especially pediatrician Tom Fitch, M.D., gynecologist Gene Rudd, M.D., and adolescent specialist David Spivey, M.D. Others who freely offered their time and their insights in reviewing this manuscript included the elder board at my home church, the Little Log Church in Palmer Lake, Colorado. Thanks to Pastor Chris Taylor, Pastor John Blase, Steve Dail, and Doug Jenkins. All of these men have helped me write a book that is medically reliable and biblically sound.

I appreciate Rick Christian and Lee Hough at Alive Communications, literary agents par excellence, who not only represent me but have become special friends. Thanks also to my longtime attorney, legal counselor, and friend Ned McLeod.

I owe a special acknowledgment to Dr. James Dobson. As a young parent and husband, I depended on Dr. Dobson's practical advice on raising adolescents via his books and video series.

I'm thankful for Bill and Jane Judge, the experienced mentors Barb and I relied on as we nurtured our teens. The two of them, who had nurtured five highly healthy teens, counseled us and answered our questions. Thanks also to Jerry and Jennifer Adamson, Don and Pauline Rinkus, Nancy Franklin, and Sam and Nancy Cunningham, who are dear friends and who were raising their teens at the same time we were. Without their support, love, and prayers, I'm not sure Barb and I would have survived the teen years! They all helped us become healthier parents and a healthier family.

I want to acknowledge my best friend of more than forty-seven years and my wife of thirty-one years, Barb. All she's done and sacrificed to make it possible for me to write cannot be overstated. Barb, I love you.

To Kate and Scott, the two teens God gave to Barb and me, I owe my gratitude for allowing me to share your stories. In many ways they were my most accomplished professors in the school of parenting highly healthy children. Now I'm the grateful father of two highly healthy young adults. Being their father is one of the most wonderful privileges of my life.

Finally, I'm grateful to God for allowing me to serve him through writing. My deepest prayer is that this work will bring glory to him and his health principles to you.

Notes

Chapter 1: What Is a Highly Healthy Teen?

28: *"The LORD gives strength"*: Psalm 29:11.

28: *"Love and faithfulness"*: Psalm 85:10.

28: *"a heart at peace"*: Proverbs 14:30.

29: *"A cheerful heart"*: Proverbs 17:22.

29: *"For day and night"*: Psalm 32:3–4.

29: *"Dear friend, I pray"*: 3 John 2.

29: *"Sermon on the Mount"*: See Matthew 5:3–12; Luke 6:20–26.

30: *"our teens will simply be less healthy"*: A few verses that support this statement: Proverbs 17:22; Matthew 5:3–12; 6:33; 16:26; Luke 6:20–26; 1 Corinthians 11:29–30; 3 John 2.

31: *"Jesus grew in wisdom"*: Luke 2:52.

33: *"For physical training"*: 1 Timothy 4:8.

33: *"promise an abundant life"*: See John 10:10.

Chapter 2: Assessing Your Teen's Health

45: *"For married parents of adopted children"*: In my book *God's Design for the Highly Healthy Child*, I discuss the possibility that adopted children are at greater risk than biological children for not becoming highly healthy (see Walt Larimore, M.D., *God's Design for the Highly Healthy Child* [Grand Rapids: Zondervan, 2004], 183–84).

Chapter 3: We Have Ignition: Preparing for the Puberty Years

57: *"Lintball Leo's"*: Walt Larimore, *Lintball Leo's Not-So-Stupid Questions About Your Body* (Grand Rapids: Zondervan, 2003).

63: *A Chicken's Guide"*: Dr. Kevin Leman and Kathy Flores Bell, *A Chicken's Guide to Talking Turkey with Your Kids about Sex* (Grand Rapids: Zondervan, 2004).

64: *"Precocious puberty"*: See the article on "Precocious Puberty" (online at www.ehendrick.org/healthy/001082.htm). You can learn more about precocious puberty at www.kidshealth.org/parent/medical/sexual/precocious .html; www.drgreene .com/21_356.html; and www.pediatrics.about.com/library/weekly/aa090900.htm.

66: *Child Trends Report"*: Child Trends (www.childtrends.org) is a nonprofit, nonpartisan children's research organization that collects and analyzes data. This information comes from the 2002 report.

67: *"Institute for Youth Development"*: Cited in Kathryn Hooks, "'Hands-on' Love"; can be viewed on the Web at www.cwfa.org/articles/4243/BLI/dot commentary/.

67: *"Journal of Family Issues"*: Hee-Og Sim and Sam Vuchinich, "The Declining Effects of Family Stressors on Antisocial Behavior from Childhood to Adolescence and Early Adulthood," *Journal of Family Issues* 17 (1996): 408–27.

67–68: *"The Parent Trap"*: Cited in William Mattox Jr., "The Parent Trap," *Policy Review* 55 (Winter 1991): 10; can be viewed on the Web at www.heritage .org/research/features/ISSUES/98/chap6.html#pgfId=1008060.

68: *"1,500 schoolchildren"*: Reported in Hooks, "'Hands-on' Love."

68: *"Preparing for Adolescence"*: See Dr. James Dobson, *Preparing for Adolescence*, updated ed. (Ventura, Calif.: Regal, 1999).

69: *"love languages"*: See Gary Chapman, *The Five Love Languages of Teenagers* (Chicago: Northfield, 2000), 45–117.

70: *Richard Swenson"*: Richard Swenson, *Margin: Restoring Emotional, Physical, Financial, and Time Reserves to Overloaded Lives* (Colorado Springs: NavPress, 1992).

Chapter 4: You're Two-Thirds of the Way There

78: *"The leading cause of death"*: Reported in National Highway Traffic Safety Administration, "Teen Crash Statistics"; can be viewed on the Web at www .nhtsa.dot.gov/people/injury/newdriver/SaveTeens/append_c.html.

78: *"Teens are four times more likely"*: Reported in Centers for Disease Control, "Teen Drivers: Fact Sheet"; can be viewed on the Web at www.cdc.gov/ ncipc/factsheets/teenmvh.htm.

84: *"Tanner Classification"*: Information in this section is adapted from J. Geoff Malta, "Five Stages of Puberty - Guys?"; can be viewed on the Web at www.puberty101.com/p_pubguys.shtml.

88: *"Tanner Classification"*: Information in this section is adapted from J. Geoff Malta, "Five Stages of Puberty - Girls?"; can be viewed on the Web at www .puberty101.com/p_pubgirls.shtml.

90: *"amount of pubic hair increases"*: See Barb Durso, M.D., "Girls and Puberty"; can be viewed on the Web at www.keepkidshealthy.com/development/ puberty_girls.html.

92: *"There are many good books"*: Karen Gravelle and Jennifer Gravelle, *The Period Book* (New York: Walker, 1996; Robie H. Harris, *It's Perfectly Normal* (Cambridge, Mass.: Candlewick, 1996).

93: *"People of both genders"*: Reported in Howard J. DeMonaco, "Debating the Use of Growth Hormone in Healthy But Short Children" (June 20, 2003); can be viewed on the Web at www.intelihealth.com/IH/ihtIH/WSIH W000/333 /349/365782.html.

93: *"Other researchers believe"*: Reported in Scott Adams, "Short Children Too Often Viewed as Handicapped, UF Researchers Say" (December 11, 1996); can be viewed on the Web at www.napa.ufl.edu/oldnews/short.htm.

94–95: *"Teen Assessment Project"*: See University of Minnesota Extension Services, "Living with Your Teenager: Understanding Physical Changes"; can be viewed on the Web at http://cecommerce.uwex.edu/pdfs/NCR118.PDF.

95: *"Here are some tips"*: Adapted from "Physical Changes," http://www.tipson
teens.org/topics/physical.html.

Chapter 5: Finding the Right Examination Room

102: *"board certified"*: The four specialists who most often provide care for teens
are *family physicians* (who should be board certified by the American Board
of Family Practice), *pediatricians* (American Board of Pediatrics), *internists*
(American Board of Internal Medicine), and *obstetrician/gynecologists* (American College of Obstetrics and Gynecology). There is also a new subspecialty
board for adolescent medicine; this certification is only available to those
physicians who are board certified in family practice, pediatrics, internal
medicine, or emergency medicine. This is called a Certificate of Added Qualification (CAQ) in Adolescent Medicine.

107: *"Centers for Disease Control"*: See www.cdc.gov/nip/recs/teen-schedule
.htm#chart.

107: *"Highly Healthy Child"*: See Walt Larimore, M.D., *God's Design for the
Highly Healthy Child* (Grand Rapids: Zondervan, 2004), 67–73.

107: *"Immunization Action Coalition"*: Information can be viewed at www.immu-
nize.org/catg.d/4038myth.htm. See Paul A. Offit, M.D., and Louis M. Bell,
M.D., *Vaccines: What Every Parent Should Know*, 2nd ed. (New York: IDG
Books, 1999). Topics include how vaccines are made and how they work,
practical tips about vaccines, vaccine myths, disease-specific information,
travel vaccines for children, and combination vaccines. This valuable
resource is a must-read for parents and those who immunize!

108–9: *"Testicular Cancer Resource Center"*: See www.tcrc.acor.org/tcexam.html.

111: *"Testicular Cancer Resource Center"*: See www.tcrc.acor.org/tcprimer.html.

114: *"80 percent of breast cancers"*: Well-Connected report, "Breast Cancer"; can
be viewed on the Web at www.reutershealth.com/wellconnected/doc06
.html.

Chapter 6: The Cut Look and Cutting Looks

118: *"abuse of oral or injectable anabolic steroids"*: National Institute on Drug
Abuse, "Community Drug Alert Bulletin—Anabolic Steriods"; can be
viewed on the Web at www.nida.nih.gov/ResearchReports/Steroids/Anabolic
Steroids.html.

119: *"roid rage"*: See Steven Stocker, "Study Provides Additional Evidence That
High Steroid Doses Elicit Psychiatric Symptoms in Some Men (aka roid
rage)"; can be viewed on the Web at www.steroids.org/psychiatric.htm.

119: *"Monitoring the Future"*: See L. D. Johnston, P. M. O'Malley, and J. G. Bach-
man, *Monitoring the Future: National Survey Results on Drug Use, 1975-2002,
Volume 1: Secondary School Students* (Bethesda, Md.: National Institute on
Drug Abuse, 2003).

119: *"percentage of twelfth graders"*: See National Institute on Drug Abuse, "Community Drug Alert Bulletin—Anabolic Steroids"; can be viewed on the
Web at www.nida.nih.gov/SteroidAlert/SteroidAlert.html.

119: *"Institute on Drug Abuse"*: See www.nida.nih.gov/ResearchReports/Steroids/AnabolicSteroids.html.

121: *"ConsumerLab.com"*: Reported in Walter L. Larimore and Dónal P. O'Mathúna, "Quality Assessment Programs for Dietary Supplements," *Annals of Pharmacotherapy* 37:6 (June 2003): 893–98; can be viewed on the Web at www.hwbooks.com/pdf/10.1345-aph.1D031.pdf.

121: *"Alternative Medicine"*: See Dónal O'Mathúna, Ph.D., and Walt Larimore, M.D., *Alternative Medicine: The Christian Handbook* (Grand Rapids: Zondervan, 2001).

122: *"prevalence of obesity among children"*: See Andrew Stern, "Obesity Takes Emotional Toll on Teens" (Chicago: Reuters Health, August 11, 2003); can be viewed on the Web at www.sandia.gov/health/update/20030811elin023.html. See also Brad Dorfman, "Parents Blame Selves for Children's Obesity" (Chicago: Reuters Health, August 11, 2003); can be viewed on the Web at www.preventdisease.com/news/articles/parents_blame_selves_childrens_obesity.shtml.

122–23: *"ACNielsen survey"*: See Dorfman, "Parents Blame Selves for Children's Obesity."

123: *"[Parents] can create an environment"*: Cited in Steve Jordahl, "Obese Kids Lose Weight When Parents Help" (Colorado Springs: Family News in Focus, August 15, 2003); can be viewed on the Web at http://dvlp.family.org/cforum/fnif/news/a0027365.cfm.

124: *"University of California researchers"*: See Jeffrey B. Schwimmer, Tasha M. Burwinkle, and James W. Varni, "Health-Related Quality of Life of Severely Obese Children and Adolescents," *Journal of the American Medical Association* 289:14 (April 9, 2003): 1813–19; can be viewed on the Web at www.durhamhealthpartners.org/pdfs/summit03/quality_life.pdf.

124: *"University of Minnesota study"*: See Marla E. Eisenberg, Dianne Neumark-Sztainer, and Mary Story, "Associations of Weight-Based Teasing and Emotional Well-being Among Adolescents," *Archives of Pediatrics and Adolescent Medicine* 157 (August 2003): 733–38; see also the *Archives* Journals news release, "Adolescents Teased About Their Weight May Be More Likely to Report Suicidal Thoughts and Suicide Attempts" (August 11, 2003); can be viewed on the Web at http://pubs.ama-assn.org/media/2003a/0811.dtl#teased.

125: *"Body Mass Index chart"*: The Centers for Disease Control has an excellent BMI chart with valuable explanations at www.cdc.gov/nccdphp/dnpa/bmi/bmi-for-age.htm, or you can visit the National Institutes for Health website to view the chart reproduced on page 126 (www.nhlbi.nih.gov/guidelines/obesity/bmi_tbl.pdf).

125: *"Centers for Disease Control"*: Reported in Keith Mulvihill, "CDC Makes Dire Diabetes Prediction for U.S. Children" (New Orleans: Reuters Health, June 16, 2003); can be viewed on the Web at www.drbobmartin.com/2003k_06_13news05.html.

128: *"fewer than 1 percent of teens"*: Reported in Julie Stafford, "Chew on This"; can be viewed on the Web at www.healthwell.com/delicious-online/ D_backs /Jan_99/healthbites.cfm?path=hw.

128: *"98 percent of American high schools"*: Reported in Elizabeth Becker and Marian Burros, "Eat Your Vegetables? Only at a Few Schools," *New York Times,* January 13, 2003, A1.

129: *"1998 survey"*: Reported in Judy McBride, "Today's Kids Are Eating More" (Agricultural Research Service, August 11, 2000); can be viewed on the Web at www.ars.usda.gov/is/pr/2000/000811.htm.

129: *"sixty-five gallons of soft drinks"*: Reported in "For Your Health: Facts Every Mother Should Know about Kids and Obesity"; can be viewed on the Web at www.rallieonhealth.com/facts.php.

129–30: *"national survey of parents"*: Reported in Steve Farkas, Jean Johnson, and Ann Duffett, *A Lot Easier Said Than Done: Parents Talk about Raising Children in Today's America* (New York: Public Agenda, 2002), 20; can be viewed on the Web at www.publicagenda.org/specials/parents/parents.htm.

134: *"Harvard Medical School study"*: See Matthew W. Gillman et al., "Family Dinner and Diet Quality Among Older Children and Adolescents," *Archives of Family Medicine* 9:3 (March 2000): 235–40. See also "Children Eat Healthier If They Sit Down to Dinner," (New York: Reuters Health, March 15, 2000); can be viewed on the Web at www.vegsource.com/talk/ science/messages /955.html.

134: *"American Psychological Association"*: Reported in B. S. Bowden and J. M. Zeisz, "Supper's On! Adolescent Adjustment and Frequency of Family Mealtimes" (paper presented to 105th Annual Meeting of the American Psychological Association); see article on the Web at www.sciencedaily.com/ releases/1997/08/970821001329.htm.

134: *"National Merit Scholars"*: Reported in Mimi Knight, "The Family that Eats Together . . . ," *Christian Parenting Today* (January/February 2002); can be viewed on the Web at www.christianitytoday.com/cpt/2002/001/3.30.html.

136: *"Harvard researchers"*: See Walter C. Willett, M.D., *Eat, Drink, and Be Healthy: The Harvard Medical School Guide to Healthy Eating* (New York: Free Press, 2002).

137: *"Some researchers now recommend"*: Reported in Scott Gottlieb, "Men Should Eat Nine Servings of Fruit and Vegetables a Day," *BMJ* 326 (May 10, 2003): 1003; can be viewed on the Web at http://bmj.com/cgi/content/ full/326 /7397/1003/a?etoc.

138: *"Katherine Tucker"*: Reported in Valerie Green, "Introducing the New Food Pyramid: Researchers Believe There Is a Better Way to Eat," *Tufts Nutrition* (October 1, 2001); can be viewed on the Web at www.nutrition.tufts .edu/consumer/matters/2001-10-01.html.

141: *"Center for Mental Health Services"*: Reported in National Mental Health Information Center, "Eating Disorders"; can be viewed on the Web at www .mentalhealth.org/publications/allpubs/ken98-0047/default.asp.

141: *"eight million people"*: Reported in Phillipa Jane Hay, "Eating Disorders,"
      Patient Guide (May 9, 2001); can be viewed on the Web at http://praxis.md/
      index.asp?page=bhg_report&article_id=BHG01PS20&section=report.

Chapter 7: For Appearance' Sake

148: *"Harris Interactive Poll"*: Reported in Joy Marie Sever, "A Third of Ameri-
      cans With Tattoos Say They Make Them Feel More Sexy" (The Harris Poll
      #58, October 8, 2003); can be viewed on the Web at www.harrisinteractive
      .com/harris_poll/index.asp?PID=407.

157: *"one out of every 200 teen girls"*: Reported in PageWise, "What Is Self Muti-
      lation and Other Self Abusive Behaviors?"; can be viewed on the Web at
      http://ct.essortment.com/whatisselfmut_rfyb.htm.

157: *"Centre for Suicide Research"*: Reported in Martin Winkler, "Prevalence of
      Cutting, Self-Mutilation and Self-Harm Among Teenagers"; can be viewed
      on the Web at http://web4health.info/en/answers/border-selfharm-prev
      .htm. See Keith Hawton et al., "Deliberate Self Harm in Adolescents: Self
      Report Survey in Schools in England," *BMJ* 325 (2002): 1207–11; can be
      viewed on the Web at www.pubmedcentral.nih.gov/articlerender.fcgi?
      artid=135492&rendertype =abstract.

158: *"American Society of Plastic Surgeons"*: Reported in Focus on Your Family's
      Health, "Cosmetic Surgery for Teens"; can be viewed on the Web at
      http://health.family.org/teens/articles/a0000316.html.

158: *"number of teenage girls"*: Reported in CBSNews.com, "Shaping the Perfect
      Teenager (June 22, 2000); can be viewed on the Web at www.cbsnews.com/
      stories/1999/05/25/48hours/main48474.shtml.

Chapter 8: The ABC's—and D's—of Nurturing Your Teen

166: *"Hillary Rodham Clinton"*: Cited in Dr. James Dobson, *Bringing Up Boys*
      (Wheaton, Ill.: Tyndale House, 2001), 219.

167: *"Michael Reagan"*: "Michael Reagan: Overcoming the Past," interview with
      Dr. James Dobson, Focus on the Family radio program (September 24,
      2003).

171: *"Edward M. Hallowell"*: Edward M. Hallowell, M.D., *The Childhood Roots
      of Adult Happiness* (New York: Ballantine, 2002), 62.

173: *"From Dr. Dobson's writings"*: Adapted from James C. Dobson, Ph.D., *The
      Strong-Willed Child* (Wheaton, Ill.: Tyndale House, 1978); see article on
      the Web at www.family.org/pplace/toddlers/a0000024.cfm.

173: *"Dr. Dobson suggests"*: James C. Dobson, Ph.D., *Complete Marriage and
      Family Home Reference Guide* (Wheaton, Ill.: Tyndale House, 2000).

174: *"Diana Baumrind"*: See Diana Baumrind, "The influence of parenting style
      on adolescent competence and substance use," *Journal of Early Adolescence*
      11:1 (1991): 56–95; see article on the Web at www.vtaide.com/png/ERIC/
      Parenting-Styles.htm.

174: *"parenting style captures two important elements"*: Reported in E. E. Maccoby
      and J. A. Martin, "Socialization in the context of the family: Parent-child

interaction," in P. H. Mussen (ed.) and E. M. Hetherington (vol. ed.), *Handbook of Child Psychology: Vol. 4. Socialization, Personality, and Social Development*, 4th ed. (New York: Wiley, 1983), 1–101.

174: *"Parental responsiveness"*: Baumrind, "The influence of parenting style," 61–62.

175: *"Researchers have found"*: Reported in Robin F. Goodman and Anita Gurian, "Parental Styles/Children's Temperaments: The Match"; can be viewed on the Web at www.aboutourkids.org/aboutour/articles/parentingstyles.html.

178: *"I agree with the experts"*: See M. A. Straus, "Spanking and the Making of a Violent Society," *Pediatrics* 98 (1996): 837–42; M. A. Straus, D. B. Sugarman, and J. Giles-Sims, "Spanking by Parents and Subsequent Antisocial Behavior of Children," *Archives of Pediatrics and Adolescent Medicine* 151 (1997): 761–67.

Chapter 9: Escape into Ecstasy

184: *"Studies indicate that even the first dose"*: Reported in Donna Leinwand and Gary Fields, "Feds Crack Down on Ecstasy," *USA Today* (April 19, 2000); can be viewed on the Web at www.billstclair.com/911timeline/2000/usatoday 041900.html.

186: *"Young people who consider religion"*: Office of National Drug Control Policy, "Drug Czar, White House & Faith Communities Join to Prevent Teen Marijuana Use" (July 10, 2003); can be viewed on the Web at http://usinfo .state.gov/usa/faith/pr071103.htm.

186: *"1999 Gallup Poll"*: Reported in "Faith: TheAntiDrug.com's Resource for Faith Leaders"; can be viewed on the Web at www.theantidrug.com/faith/ index.asp.

187: *"Detective Scott Perkins"*: Cited in Sara Trollinger, *Unglued and Tattooed* (Washington, D.C.: LifeLine, 2001), 33–34.

187–88: *"We had never heard of huffing"*: Cited in Stephanie Stapleton, "Is Your Patient (or Child) Abusing Inhalants?" *AM News* (April 9, 2001); can be viewed on the Web at www.ama-assn.org/amednews/2001/04/09/hlsc0409 .htm.

188: *"one teen in five has tried sniffing"*: Reported in Deborah Zabarenko, "Alert: 1st-time Sniffers Can Die," *Detroit Free Press* (March 16, 2001); can be viewed on the Web at www.freep.com/news/health/huff16_20010316.htm.

188: *"National Household Survey"*: Reported in Stapleton, "Is Your Patient (or Child) Abusing Inhalants?"; see also Office of National Drug Control Policy, "Inhalants"; can be viewed on the Web at www.whitehousedrugpolicy .gov/drugfact/inhalants/.

188: *"National Inhalant Prevention Coalition"*: Reported in National Inhalant Prevention Coalition, "About Inhalants"; can be viewed on the Web at www.inhalants.org/about.htm.

190: *"Solomon"*: Proverbs 5:23 (The Message).

190: *"Young people are prone"*: Proverbs 22:15 (The Message)

190: *"Partnership for a Drug-Free America"*: "#1 Hypocrite," *Parade* (April 11, 2004), 8.

190: *"the Bible says"*: See Romans 13:13; Ephesians 5:18.

192: *"stressed-out, bored teens who receive $25"*: Reported in Sue Pleming, "Stressed Teens with Money at Risk for Drug Use" (Washington: Reuters Health, August 19, 2003).

194: *"according to a 2003 study"*: Reported in Pleming, "Stressed Teens with Money at Risk for Drug Use."

195: *"Youth Risk Survey"*: Reported in "Youth Risk Behavior Surveillance Data - 2001,"; can be viewed on the Web at http://smhp.psych.ucla.edu/qf/suicide_qt/yrbsdata.pdf.

195: *"Bipolar disorder"*: Reported in "Stanford Study of Genetics of Bipolar Disease May Help Predict Disease in Kids"; can be viewed on the Web at www.stanfordhospital.com/newsEvents/newsReleases/2003/03/biplarKids.html.

195: *"Experts say that ADHD affects"*: Reported in National Institute of Mental Health, "Attention Deficit/Hyperactivity Disorder"; can be viewed on the Web at www.kidsource.com/kidsource/content2/add.nimh.html.

196: *"Untreated teens"*: See "ADHD or ADD: Signs, Symptoms, or Subtypes"; can be viewed on the Web at www.helpguide.org/mental/adhd_add_signs_symptoms.htm.

197: *"Why A.D.H.D. Doesn't Mean Disaster"*: Dennis Swanberg and Diane Passno, with medical contributions by Walt Larimore, M.D., *Why A.D.H.D. Doesn't Mean Disaster* (Wheaton, Ill.: Tyndale House, 2003).

200: *"New Light on Depression"*: David B. Biebel, D.Min, and Harold G. Koenig, M.D., *New Light on Depression: Help, Hope, and Answers for the Depressed and Those Who Love Them* (Grand Rapids: Zondervan, 2004).

201: *"White House–sponsored survey"*: Reported in Gilbert Ross, "Rate Films with Smoking 'R' for Their Influence on Kids," *USA Today* (August 20, 2003); can be viewed on the Web at www.usatoday.com/news/opinion/editorials/2003-08-19-ross_x.htm.

201: *"Scientists from the Dartmouth Medical School"*: Reported in Ross, "Rate Films with Smoking 'R' for Their Influence on Kids."

201: *"Teens who smoke cigarettes are fourteen times"*: Reported in Cyrille Cartier, "Teen Smokers More Likely to Try Marijuana" (Washington: Reuters Health, September 16, 2003).

Chapter 10: Home Channel Network

203: *"It took forty-five years"*: Reported in "The Speed of Life: The Race for Space at the Table," *Consumer Insight*; can be viewed on the Web at www.acnielsen.com/pubs/ci/2001/q1/features/speed_life.htm.

204: *"The U.S. household average"*: Compiled by the TV-Free America; can be viewed on the Web at www.csun.edu/~vceed002/health/docs/tv&health.html.

204: *"Harris Interactive Poll from 2003"*: Reported in Brian Morrissey, "Study: Teen Use Net More Than TV"; can be viewed on the Web at www.clickz .com /news/article.php/2240141.

205: *"American Journal of Public Health"*: See L. A. Tucker and G. M. Friedman, "Television Viewing and Obesity in Adult Males," *American Journal of Public Health* 79 (April 1989): 516–18.

206: *"more than half of parents report"*: Reported in Steve Farkas, Jean Johnson, and Ann Duffett, *A Lot Easier Said Than Done: Parents Talk about Raising Children in Today's America* (New York: Public Agenda, 2002), 13.

206: *"42 percent of children ages nine to seventeen"*: Reported in Federal Trade Commission, "Appendix B: Children as Consumers of Entertainment Media: Media Usage, Marketing Behavior and Influences, and Ratings Effects," (September 1, 2000); can be viewed on the Web at www.ftc.gov/ reports/violence/Appen%20B.pdf.

206: *"One study of 450 young people"*: Reported in Dale and Karen Mason, "How much TV is too much TV?"; can be viewed on the Web at www.christian answers.net/q-eden/edn-f009.html.

207: *"UCLA researchers found"*: Reported in Roxanne Moster, "TV News Skews Viewer Perception of Threats to Life and Limb"(December 2001); can be viewed on the Web at www.ph.ucla.edu/sph/pr/newsitem120301.html.

208: *"Studies have shown"*: Reported in Dale Mason, Karen Mason, and Ken Wales, *How to Get the Best Out of TV: Before It Gets the Best of You* (Nashville: Broadman & Holman, 1996); can be viewed on the Web at www.christian answers.net/tv1/tvb-ch5.html.

209: *"children watching TV tend to burn"*: Cited in Mason, Mason, and Wales, *How to Get the Best Out of TV.*

209: *"these effects are reversible"*: Reported in Thomas N. Robinson, "Reducing Children's Television Viewing to Prevent Obesity; A Randomized Controlled Trial," *Journal of the American Medical Association* 282 (1999): 1561–67.

209: *"a nationwide, ethnically balanced survey"*: Cited in Mason, Mason, and Wales, *How to Get the Best Out of TV.*

209: *"Barbara Brock"*: Reported in Barbara J. Brock, "TV Free Families: Are They Lola Granolas, Normal Joes or High and Holy Snots?"; can be viewed on the Web at www.tvturnoff.org/brock2.htm.

212: *"Harris Interactive Poll"*: Reported in Morrissey, "Study: Teen Use Net More Than TV."

213: *"Parenting with Dignity"*: Adapted from Parenting with Dignity, "Warning Signs: Chat Rooms"; can be viewed on the Web at www.warningsigns.info/ chat_rooms_warning_signs.htm.

215: *"English playwright Thomas Dekker"*: Cited in the Quote Garden, "Quotations about Sleep"; can be viewed on the Web at www.quotegarden.com/ sleep.html.

215: *"Medical research shows"*: Reported in Rita Mullin, "Helping Sleep-Deprived Teens"; can be viewed on the Web at www.health.discovery.com/centers/ sleepdreams/basics/teens.html.

216:    *"Tired kids get lower grades"*: Reported in Barbara Kantrowitz and Karen Springen, "Why Sleep Matters," *Newsweek* (September 22, 2003); can be viewed on the Web at www.msnbc.msn.com/id/3068894/.

216:    *"survey by the National Sleep Foundation"*: Reported in National Sleep Foundation, "1998 Omnibus Sleep in America Poll"; can be viewed on the Web at www.sleepfoundation.org/publications/1998poll.cfm#1.

216:    *"In a 1999 survey"*: Reported in National Sleep Foundation, "1999 Omnibus Sleep in America Poll"; can be viewed on the Web at www.sleepfoundation .org/publications/1999poll.cfm#5.

Chapter 11: Family Matters

222:    *"David Popenoe"*: David Popenoe, *Promises to Keep* (Lanham, Md.: Rowman and Littlefield, 1996), 248.

222:    *"parental divorce"*: Reported in Jane Mauldon, "The Effects of Marital Disruption on Children's Health," *Demography* 27 (1990): 431–46.

223:    *"2002 study that reviewed"*: Reported in Rebecca O'Neill, "Experiments in Living: The Fatherless Family" (London: Civitas, September 2002); can be viewed on the Web at www.civitas.org.uk/pubs/experiments.php.

223:    *"Children from disrupted marriages"*: Reported in O'Neill, "Experiments in Living"; see also Deborah A. Dawson, "Family Structure and Children's Health and Well-being: Data from the 1988 National Health Interview Survey on Child Health," *Journal of Marriage and the Family* 53 (August 1991): 573–84.

223:    *"Children from single-parent families"*: Reported in Nicholas Zill and Charlotte A. Schoenborn, "Developmental, Learning, and Emotional Problems: Health of Our Nation's Children, United States, 1988," *Advance Data from Vital and Health Statistics*, vol. 190, publication #120 (Hyattsville, Md.: National Center for Health Statistics, November 1990).

223:    *"Judith Wallerstein"*: Reported in Judith S. Wallerstein and Sandra Blakeslee, *Second Chances: Men, Women and Children a Decade After Divorce* (Boston: Ticknor and Fields, 1989), xvii.

223:    *"Teens of divorced parents"*: Reported in O'Neill, "Experiments in Living."

225:    *"Fatherlessness is a major epidemic"*: Reported in Wade F. Horn and Tom Sylvester, *Father Facts, 4th edition* (Gaithersburg, Md: National Fatherhood Initiative, 2002); can be viewed on the Web at www.fatherhood.org/father facts /topten.htm.

225:    *"teenagers living with their biological fathers"*: Reported in O'Neill, "Experiments in Living."

225:    *"teens with involved, loving fathers"*: Reported in Horn and Sylvester, *Father Facts,* 16.

225:    *"National Fatherhood Initiative"*: Reported in Horn and Sylvester, *Father Facts,* 16.

225:    *"father love is a better predictor"*: Reported in R. P. Rohner and R. A. Veneziano, "The Importance of Father Love: History and Contemporary Evidence," *Review of General Psychology* 5:4 (December 2001): 382–405.

226: *"Mom's responsibilities can never"*: Reported in Karl Zinsmeister, "The Importance of Early Attachment," *The American Enterprise* (May/June 1998), 30.

227: *"teens are three times more likely"*: Reported in Joseph A. Califano Jr., "It's All in the Family," *America* (January 15, 2000), e2; can be viewed on the Web at www.americamagazine.org/gettext.cfm?articleTypeID=1&text ID =482&issueID=272.

227: *"The Bible indicates"*: "The LORD is slow to anger, abounding in love and forgiving sin and rebellion. Yet he does not leave the guilty unpunished; he punishes the children for the sin of the fathers to the third and fourth generation" (Numbers 14:18; see also Exodus 20:5; 34:7; Deuteronomy 5:9).

228: *"five times as likely"*: Reported in Horn and Sylvester, *Father Facts*, 16.

228: *"Single-parent moms are far more likely"*: Reported in Kersti Yllo and Murray A. Strauss, "Interpersonal Violence Among Married and Cohabiting Couples," *Family Relations* 30 (1981): 339.

229: *"Gary Richmond"*: Gary Richmond, *Successful Single Parenting: Bringing Out the Best in Your Kids* (Eugene, Ore.: Harvest House, 1998).

229: *"remarriage divorce rate"*: Reported in Stepfamily Association of America, "Stepfamily Facts"; can be viewed on the Web at www.saafamilies.org/faqs/index.htm.

Chapter 12: How Clear Is Your Teen's Connection?

231: *"All happy families are alike"*: Leo Tolstoy, *Anna Karenina* (New York: Penguin, 2003), 1.

232: *"Dr. Hallowell"*: Edward M. Hallowell, M.D., *The Childhood Roots of Adult Happiness* (New York: Ballantine, 2002), 62.

236: *"Do not be misled"*: 1 Corinthians 15:33.

236: *"Research shows that teens"*: Reported in J. G. Parker and S. R. Asher, "Peer Relations and Later Personal Adjustment: Are Low-Accepted Children at Risk?" *Psychological Bulletin* 102 (1987): 357.

Chapter 13: Getting All Hot and Bothered

246: *"National Institutes of Health"*: Reported in National Institutes of Health, "An Introduction to Sexually Transmitted Diseases"; can be viewed on the Web at www.niaid.nih.gov/factsheets/stdinfo.htm.

246: *"A CDC study released in 2003"*: See Kathleen A. Ethier, et al., "Adolescent women underestimate their susceptibility to sexually transmitted infections," *Sexually Transmitted Infections* 79 (October 2003): 408–11; can be viewed on the Web at http://cira.med.yale.edu/events/STI_article.pdf. See also Merritt McKinney, "Many Teenage Girls Underestimate STI Risk" (New York: Reuters Health, October 15, 2003); can be viewed on the Web at http://cira.mcd.yale .edu/events/stdrisk_article.html.

247: *"An estimated 20 to 30 percent"*: Reported in Office of Technology Assessment, *Infertility: Medical and Social Changes* (Washington, D.C.: U.S. Government Printing Office, 1988), 85; can be viewed on the Web at www.wws

.princeton.edu/cgi-bin/byteserv.prl/~ota/disk2/1988/8822/882207.PDF. See also Office of Women's Health, "Sexually Transmitted Diseases: An Overview for Women"; can be viewed on the Web at www.thebody.com/cdc/stdover view.html.

248: *"91 percent of sexually active teens"*: Reported in Jennifer Warner, "Home Alone and Having Sex," *WebMD* (December 2, 2002); can be viewed on the Web at http://content.health.msn.com/content/article/54/65226.htm. See also D. A. Cohen, et al., "When and Where Do Youths Have Sex? The Potential Role of Adult Supervision," *Pediatrics* 110:6 (December 2002): e66; can be viewed on the Web at http://pediatrics.aappublications.org/cgi/content/full /110/6/e66.

248: *"A study by the Urban Institute"*: Reported in "Premarital Sex and Teens," *Rocky Mountain Family Council Advisor* (Spring 1999); can be viewed on the Web at www.rmfc.org/adv99sp.html.

248: *"A research brief filed by"*: Reported in "Science Says: Where and When Teens First Have Sex," *Child Trends* (June 2003); can be viewed on the Web at www.teenpregnancy.org/works/pdf/sciencesayswherewhen.pdf.

249: *"Research has shown that parents"*: Reported in Sharon D. White and Richard R. DeBlassie, "Adolescent Sexual Behavior," *Adolescence* 27:105 (1992): 183–91; see William Gaultiere, "Sexual Purity in an R-Rated Culture'" can be viewed on the Web at http://newhopenow.org/counselors/ce/sex.purity .html.

254: *"According to a 1999 study undertaken"*: Reported in Alan Guttmacher Institute, "Trend toward Abstinence-Only Sex Ed Means Many U.S. Teenagers Are Not Getting Vital Messages about Contraception," News Release; can be viewed on the Web at www.agi-usa.org/pubs/archives/newsrelease3205 .html.

254: *"According to a 2003 CDC survey"*: Reported in North Carolina Family Policy Council, "CDC Report Finds Teen Sexual Activity Still Too High" (June 3, 2004); can be viewed on the Web at www.ncfpc.org/stories/040603s1 .html.

260: *"Every Young Man's Battle"*: Stephen Arterburn and Fred Stoeker, with Mike Yorkey, *Every Young Man's Battle* (Colorado Springs: WaterBrook, 2002), 109.

260–61: *"Arterburn and Stoeker recommend"*: Arterburn and Stoeker, *Every Young Man's Battle*, 119.

261: *"Dr. James Dobson"*: Adapted from Dr. James Dobson, *Complete Marriage and Family Home Reference Guide* (Wheaton, Ill.: Tyndale House, 2000); can be viewed on the Web at www.focusonyourchild.com/develop/art1/A0000553 .html.

262: *"I'm convinced from people"*: Cited in Kent Paris, "The Seduction of Our Youth: Christian Parents Are Discovering It CAN Happen Here"; can be viewed on the Web at www.exodus-international.org/library_Society_09 .shtml. See also National Association for Research & Therapy of Homosexuality, "Prominent Psychiatrist Announces New Study Results: 'Some Gays can Change,'" Press Release (May 9, 2001); can be viewed on the Web at www.narth.com/docs /spitzerrelease.html.

262: *"There is evidence that change"*: Robert L. Spitzer, "Can Some Gay Men and Lesbians Change Their Sexual Orientation? 200 Participants Reporting a Change from Homosexual to Heterosexual Orientation," *Archives of Sexual Behavior* 32:5 (October 2003): 403–17.

263: *"Dr. Nicolosi was asked to share findings"*: Joseph Nicolosi and Linda Ames Nicolosi, *A Parent's Guide to Preventing Homosexuality* (Downers Grove, Ill.: InterVarsity Press, 2002).

263: *"Dr. Nicolosi has agreed"*: Adapted from Dr. Joseph Nicolosi, "Is This Really Good for Kids?"; can be viewed on the Web at www.family.org/cforum/ teachersmag/features/a0013018.cfm.

Chapter 14: Building on the Solid Rock

270: *"International Bible Society survey"*: Reported in Howard Culbertson, "When Americans Become Christians"; can be viewed on the Web at http://home .snu.edu/~hculbert.fs/ages.htm.

270: *"Barna Research Group conducted"*: Reported in Culbertson, "When Americans Become Christians."

270: *"Faithful Parents, Faithful Kids"*: Greg Johnson and Mike Yorkey, *Faithful Parents, Faithful Kids* (Wheaton, Ill.: Tyndale House, 1993).

270: *"list the top ten"*: Johnson and Yorkey, *Faithful Parents, Faithful Kids*, 237-38.

271: *"another Barna Research survey found"*: Reported in "Teenagers," *Barna Research Online*; can be viewed on the Web at www.barna.org/cgi-bin/Page Category.asp?CategoryID=37.

273: *"found that religious belief among teens"*: Reported in John C. Thomas, "Root Causes of Juvenile Violence: Part 2 Spiritual Emptiness"; can be viewed on the Web at www.focusonyourchild.com/develop/art1/A0001084.html.

274: *"facts from the Barna Group"*: "Teenagers," *Barna Research Online*.

274: *"we display the spiritual fruit"*: See Galatians 5:22–23. This can also be called "positive spirituality" because of the positive impact it has on people, their families, and society. See W. L. Larimore, M. Parker, and M. Crowther, "Should Clinicians Incorporate Positive Spirituality into Their Practices? What Does the Evidence Say?" *Annals of Behavioral Medicine* 24:1 (2002): 69–73.

274: *"research shows that highly healthy"*: Reported in Harold G. Koenig, Michael E. McCullough, and David B. Larson, *Handbook of Religion and Health* (New York: Oxford Univ. Press, 2001) 78–94.

275: *"A teen named Cassie Bernall"*: See Matt Labash, "Do You Believe in God? Yes," *The Weekly Standard* 32 (May 10, 1999), 23.

275–76: *"embraced the dark elements"*: Reported in Erin Emery, "Video, Poems Foreshadowed Day of Disaster," *Denver Post*, April 22, 1999, 10A.

276: *"spiritual foundation is associated with"*: Reported in A. W. Braam et al., "Religious Involvement and Depression in Older Dutch Citizens," *Social Psychiatry and Psychiatric Epidemiology* 32 (1997): 284–91.

276: *"What on earth am I here for?"*: See Rick Warren, *The Purpose-Driven Life* (Grand Rapids: Zondervan, 2002), 15.

277: *"Energizing Your Teenager's Faith"*: Jay Kesler, *Energizing Your Teenager's Faith* (Loveland, Colo.: Group, 1990).

279: *"2001 survey conducted by the Barna Group"*: Barna Updates, "Americans Are Most Likely to Base Truth on Feelings" (February 12, 2002); can be viewed on the Web at www.barna.org/FlexPage.aspx?Page=BarnaUpdate &BarnaUpdateID=106.

280–81: *"Pastor Rick Warren"*: Warren, *The Purpose-Driven Life*, 65–66.

283: *"For physical training"*: 1 Timothy 4:8.

Chapter 15: Into the Clubhouse Turn

288: *"U.S. Census Bureau"*: Reported in Robert Mills and Shailesh Bhandari, "Health Insurance Coverage in the United States: 2002"; can be viewed on the Web at www.census.gov/prod/2003pubs/p60-223.pdf.

290: *"Research is showing"*: Reported in Barnabas Counseling Center, "Premarital Counseling"; can be viewed on the Web at www.barnabascounseling.com/ templates/cla21gr/details.asp?id=26228&PID=129038.

291–92: *"psalmist wrote this about children"*: Psalm 127:3–5 NASB.

Subject Index

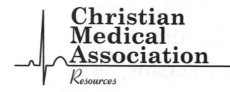

Christian Medical Association
Resources

Medically reliable . . . biblically sound. That's the rock-solid promise of this series offered by Zondervan in partnership with the Christian Medical Association. Each book in this series is not only written by fully credentialed, experienced doctors but is also fully reviewed by an objective board of qualified doctors to ensure its reliability. Because when your health is at stake, you can't settle for anything less than the whole and accurate truth.

Integrating your faith and health can improve your physical well-being and even extend your life, as you gain insights into the interconnection of health and faith—a relationship largely overlooked by secular science. Benefit from the cutting-edge knowledge of respected medical experts as they help you make health care decisions consistent with your beliefs. Their sound biblical analysis of emerging treatments and technologies equips you to protect yourself from seemingly harmless—yet spiritually, ethically, or medically unsound—options and then to make the healthiest choices possible.

Through this series, you can draw from both the knowledge of science and the wisdom of God's Word in addressing your medical ethics decisions and in meeting your health care needs.

Founded in 1931, the Christian Medical Association helps thousands of doctors minister to their patients by imitating the Great Physician, Jesus Christ. Christian Medical Association members provide a Christian voice on medical ethics to policy makers and the media, minister to needy patients on medical missions around the world, evangelize and disciple students on more than 90 percent of the nation's medical school campuses, and provide educational and inspirational resources to the church.

To learn more about Christian Medical Association ministries and resources on health care and ethical issues, browse the website (www.christian medicalassociation.org) or call toll-free at 1-888-231-2637.

"Dear friend, I pray that you may enjoy good health and that all may go well with you, even as your soul is getting along well" (3 John 2).

God's Design for the Highly Healthy Person

Walt Larimore, M.D., with Traci Mullins

A must-have resource for pursuing wellness, coping with illness, and developing a plan to care for your health needs. Learn how to assess your health, fix the "spoke" that's broke, and benefit from immediate action for improving your life and health.

God's Design for the Highly Healthy Person is like having your very own health mentor to guide you in your total health picture, from treating illness and navigating the health care system to developing a proactive approach to vibrant health.

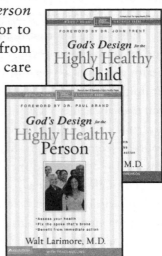

Softcover: 0-310-26279-8

God's Design for the Highly Healthy Child

Walt Larimore, M.D., with Stephen and Amanda Sorenson

You want the best for your child, especially when it comes to his or her health. You can cut through popular misconceptions and discover the surprising and proven connections between a child's physical, emotional, relational and spiritual health.

No matter what the obstacles, your child can become more highly healthy. *God's Design for the Highly Healthy Child* will teach you, in very practical ways, how to assess your child's health, fix the "spoke" that's broke, and follow advice that can make a difference in your child's health immediately.

Softcover: 0-310-26283-6